MW00978076

idealplan

Your 12 Week *Delicious* Nutrition Guide for **Maximum** Fat Loss

Lindsey Mathews
David Meine

The **IdealPlan** *solves all the problems* of weight loss:

Unbelievably simple. The biggest secret to fat loss is eating the right foods, in the right calorie amounts, with the right ratio of proteins, carbs and fats. Don't panic: we've done all of this for you in the IdealPlan.

Tastes delicious. Losing weight doesn't require torturing your taste buds. The IdealPlan is five flavorful meals and snacks every day, including two smooth and yummy IdealShakes to satisfy your sweet tooth.

Keeps you full for hours. Hunger is the enemy of weight loss (and ironically, most diets leave you that way). But with frequent meals and the powerful craving-crusher Slendesta®, you'll never go hungry on the IdealPlan.

Gives you energy. Balanced nutrition spread across five meals a day lets you trade those energy dips (that make you want to reach for a soda and a candy bar) for sustained energy all day long.

More convenient than fast food. It doesn't get quicker than unwrapping an IdealBar or blending up a smoothie with IdealShake! And your other meals and snacks on the Plan can be prepped together just once a week.

ACKNOWLEDGEMENTS

Everyone on the IdealShape team contributed to this book.

Special thanks to the editor, Chelsea Ratcliff, and the reviewers:
Skyler Meine, Meg Kimball, Jan Stephan, Kirsten Jackson,
Whitney Meine and Josh Lindsay.

Another special thanks to our customers,
who share their wonderful stories of transformation
and keep us inspired every day.

We dedicate this book to Tom Nightingale,
who was the inspiration for creating IdealShape.

David Meine
IdealShape, LLC
777 S Auto Mall Dr
Suite 111
American Fork, Utah 84003
www.idealshape.com
Phone: 1-800-515-0896

Published by David Meine and IdealShape, LLC March 1, 2015

First Edition
ISBN-13: 978-1-5114-6684-4 (sc)
ISBN-13: 978-1-5173-5880-8 (color)
ISBN-10: 1511466847 (e)

© 2015 David Meine and IdealShape, LLC. All rights reserved

The views expressed in this work are solely those of the authors.
The information included in this book is for educational purposes only.
It is not intended nor implied to be a substitute for professional medical advice.

No part of this book may be reproduced, stored in a retrieval system,
or transmitted by any means without the written permission of the authors.

Because of the dynamic nature of the Internet, any web addresses
or links contained in this book may have changed since publication
and may no longer be valid.

Legal Disclaimer

The information provided in this book is for informational purposes only and is not intended as
a substitute for advice from your physician or other health care professional or any information
contained on or in any product label or packaging. You should not use the information in this
book for diagnosis or treatment of any health problem or for prescription of any medication or
other treatment. Always consult with a healthcare professional before starting any diet, exercise
program or dietary supplement. You should not stop taking any medication
without first consulting your physician.

IdealShape®, IdealShake®, IdealBar® and IdealBoost® are registered trademarks of
IdealShape, LLC. IdealPlan™ is a trademark of IdealShape, LLC. The names of actual
companies and products mentioned herein may be the trademarks of their respective owners.

CONTENTS

MEET THE EXPERTS

Lindsey Mathews is the nutritionist at IdealShape. She is a weight loss nutrition expert certified with the International Society of Sports Nutrition (CISSN), and she has more than a decade of experience with one-on-one personal training, online meal planning, exercise coaching and running a fitness boot camp.

Lindsey's broad range of coaching over the last 10 years has given her unique insight into what it takes to achieve one's ideal shape. She's also a fitness model and national-level figure competitor, and she loves the process of competing against herself and helping others strive for their ideal, as well.

As a business owner, wife and mother of three young kids, people look to Lindsey for advice from someone who's "been there done that." She discovered the right combination of nutrition and exercise strategies to create her ideal shape in the minimum amount of time, in the simplest way possible — not only her ideal shape, but also a wealth of confidence, happiness in her relationships and the energy to be a better mom.

Lindsey poured her secrets into the IdealPlan, coauthored with IdealShape CEO David Meine. She is also the creator of IdealShape's workout plans, including the IdealBody exercise component of IdealPlan.

What drives Lindsey is being able to see how a few simple, healthy lifestyle changes have helped people make amazing transformations — and she hopes you will be one of them!

MEET THE EXPERTS

David Meine is the CEO and Co-founder of IdealShape. After personally unlocking many secrets of fat loss nutrition and motivation through his own weight loss journey, he founded the company with his wife, Carla Meine, in 2003.

From the beginning, David was inspired by a desire to unite individuals with a path to achieve their ideal body, lasting health and the confidence to live their ideal lives. Drawing on more than 30 years of experience as a motivational speaker, David understands the mental aspects of weight loss in a way that few weight loss experts do.

Over the years David and his team have worked to develop delicious, high-quality nutritional weight loss products that pave the way for a successful transformation. Working with Lindsey Mathews, IdealShape's nutritionist, he then created a meal plan and guide called the IdealPlan. With the plan, they've been able to show hundreds of thousands of IdealShape customers how to use the company's products as part of a complete weight loss plan for life-changing results.

David wrote the IdealMind workbook that is a helpful companion to the IdealPlan. He is the author of three more weight loss books: Diet Chaos, Think: Use Your Mind to Shrink Your Waistline, and 3-Hour Fat Loss with Lindsey Mathews. He is passionate about providing tools and support to help people achieve their ideal shape and, more importantly, keep it. He and Carla have seven children and 13 grandchildren.

INTRODUCTION

Lindsey here. Welcome to the IdealPlan! David and I are eager to show you the keys to overcoming hunger and changing your appetite, so you can get the trim, shapely body you've always wanted... and more importantly, you'll know how to keep it!

In this complete guide, we're going to give you:

The three secrets of fat loss that are almost always overlooked in other programs (and why this leads to a 95% failure rate).

The 10 nutrition accelerators that will deliver you to your ideal shape faster.

The IdealPlan meal plan, which is tailored for your weight and gender category and shows you how to incorporate IdealShape products for maximum results.

Dozens of easy recipes, approved food lists and snack ideas.

An FAQ and check-ins to help you stay on track and modify the plan to suit your needs.

As you start to burn fat, get toned, gain confidence and have more energy, and the components of your new healthy lifestyle will click into place.

Basically, our number one goal with the IdealPlan was to solve all the problems of weight loss:

> *It's too complicated.*
>
> *It doesn't taste good.*
>
> *You're hungry all the time.*
>
> *Your energy dropped to the floor.*
>
> *You don't have time.*

The IdealPlan eliminates all of these obstacles with:

- Pre-calculated calorie and macro amounts that are an ideal baseline for your weight and gender.

- Foods that both taste delicious AND help the body burn, not store, fat.

- The perfect balance of ingredients, portions and meal times to make sure you never go hungry.

- Energizing foods throughout the day, plus healthy alternatives to sodas and sugary foods.

- Convenient meals that take little or no prep time, and are great for on the go!

It's simple: if you follow the IdealPlan, you'll reach your ideal shape and be ready to live your ideal life sooner than you ever thought possible.

But before we tell you more about the IdealPlan, let me tell you that David and I have been at this for over a decade. We've shown more than a hundred thousand people how to lose weight and achieve their ideal body shape.

But we didn't start out skinny ourselves.

Far from it.

In fact, I want to share my story with you, and I bet you'll be able to relate...

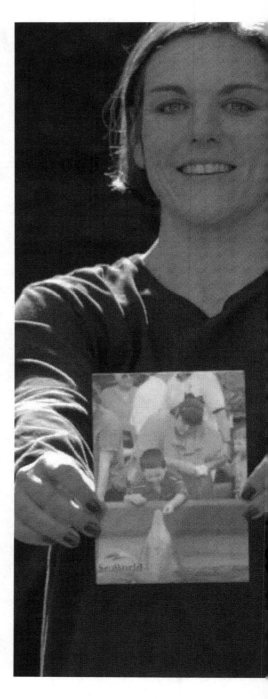

LINDSEY'S STORY

"I HAD TRIED EVERYTHING"

As a mother of three children under the age of six, my own nutrition used to be the last thing on my mind. I used to eat mindlessly all day long and wonder why I wasn't seeing results even though I "tried everything."

On more than one occasion, I saw myself in the mirror at the gym and broke down and cried. No matter how hard I worked, I couldn't shed the extra baby weight. In fact, I was gaining a few extra pounds every year. One day I sobbed to my friend, "I'm here every day and I don't even look like I exercise. What am I doing wrong?"

I was tired of sitting down to play with my kids and being reminded that all of my clothes were one size too small. Why wasn't I seeing results?

But here was the cold, hard truth: rushing around throughout the day, would pick in my kids' cereal as I was pouring it. At lunch, I was finishing the crusts of their sandwiches. And every time I walked by the pantry, I would grab a bite of something. In fact, and I'm ashamed to admit it, sometimes I even crept back into the kitchen at night, making sure my husband wasn't around, so I could sneak a few extra bites of dessert.

All the while, I felt like I was eating "pretty healthy." Now you can see why I had gradually been putting on weight despite rigorous exercise!

When I finally saw clearly that my downfall was the mindless snacking and "bites" that equaled two or three desserts a day, I looked for a solution. But being a busy wife, mother and owner of a growing fitness business, my mental energy was already stretched to the max. I needed something simple.

"I needed a clear-cut plan"

What finally helped me get my nutrition habits under control was following a black and white meal plan that I could truthfully stick with. When I tried other plans that gave me too much freedom, then I would start picking at extra food, which would turn into one bite of everything… and the whole plan would unravel again.

What's more, when I followed a plan that I didn't enjoy, the constant battle with my willpower was just too much.

But with a clear-cut plan that I actually enjoyed, I was able to flip a switch in my head and think "this

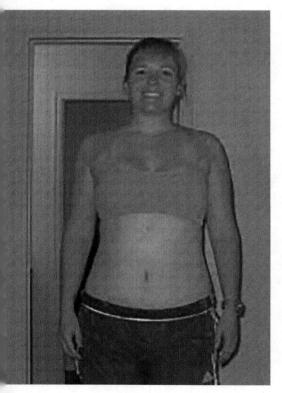

Lindsey before her ideal shape

is what I eat, don't eat anything else." Soon I didn't have to think about it at all. Having a plan gave me more freedom in my life because it wasn't exhausting my willpower.

Increasingly, I felt more in control of my cravings, and it actually made me less stressed and anxious in other areas of my life. I started to feel more calm, patient and happy. And the closer I got to my ideal shape, the more confident and strong I felt in general.

I used to pull out pictures from magazines and off the internet for my motivation. It wasn't until I reached my goals that I realized, I still didn't look like those pictures in the magazines. Instead, having a plan allowed me to become the best version of me.

This is what inspired me to start creating meal plans that would help others reach their goals. After perfecting the principles for success, I was thrilled to have the opportunity to create the IdealPlan with IdealShape.

As you can probably guess from reading my story, I LOVE food and HATE being hungry. So when

I sat down with David to create the IdealPlan, a program that real people like us could follow, our number one goal was to create a plan that was simple and clear-cut but not overly strict.

It had to be something people could stick with, and it had to include plenty of delicious foods and treats like IdealShake. It also had to be something that would deliver results without rigorous exercise, because we know that not everyone has time and not everyone is ready to start that phase of their lifestyle transformation.

AND VOILA, YOU HAVE THE IDEALPLAN

On the IdealPlan you're going to lose fat by eating frequent meals, including delicious IdealShakes, roughly every three hours. You're not going to starve yourself to the point that you're racing to the fast food drive-thru for a big greasy burger or finishing off your kids' food just because it's in front of you (like I used to do).

You're not going to feel deprived, only to find yourself hiding from your spouse in the cupboard at night with uncontrollable cravings (like I also used to do).

Instead of making your cravings stronger, you'll be indulging them with five flavorful meals a day, plus weekly "cheats." And between meals, your body is going to be hard at work burning fat like it never has before.

On the IdealPlan you will feel satisfied and energized throughout the day. You'll probably even lower your grocery bill and reduce the time it takes to shop for and prepare food! You'll also see why WHEN you eat is just as important as WHAT you eat.

In other words, the IdealPlan is the complete opposite from almost every diet out there.

Which brings us to three "secrets" of fat loss that are so often overlooked in commercial weight loss plans. These principles are the foundation of the IdealPlan and the reason it's so powerful for shedding fat and sculpting your ideal shape. So keep reading…

THREE FAT LOSS SECRETS

It's no secret that most diets fail, but you've probably never understood why. The truth: there are three critical elements of successful fat loss that are almost always ignored in popular diet programs. In fact, weight loss "experts" aren't even aware of them.

As you'll see when you start implementing the IdealPlan, understanding these three simple principles will make the journey to your ideal shape so much easier!

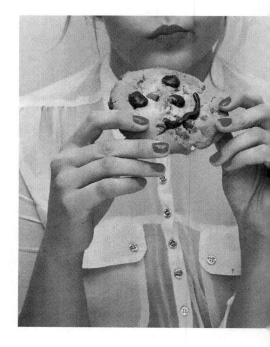

SECRET 1: HUNGER IS MOSTLY MENTAL

Have you ever been so hungry that you served yourself a huge helping or ordered extra sides at a restaurant, only to wind up full halfway through... but still eating?

Most of us would say this happens just about every day. When the idea that you're starving is guiding your forkfuls, it's easy to overestimate your hunger level and accidentally replace those

hunger pangs with an overstuffed stomach, eating more food than you need. This happens because our perception of hunger is mostly mental.

To make matters worse, hunger also causes the brain to crave unhealthy foods.

An experiment by neuroscientists at Yale and University of Southern California found that when a person is hungry, the brain lights up over high calorie, salty and sugary foods. Meanwhile, the part of the brain that governs self-control becomes less active when we're hungry.

You can see how getting really hungry is a recipe for overeating and eating all the wrong foods. And this is exactly where most diets put you.

The key to keeping your brain in sync with what your body needs? Staying satisfied and out of that hunger danger zone altogether.

SECRET 2:
INDULGE IN TREATS

Yes, you read that right. Not only is getting really hungry counter-productive, but so is depriving yourself of delicious foods and never having your favorite treats to look forward to.

And really, let's be honest. Few of us are ACTUALLY depriving ourselves when we go on a diet. More likely, we're having bites, licks and tastes (or as I like to call them, "BLTs") of everything we come across, just to get our fix.

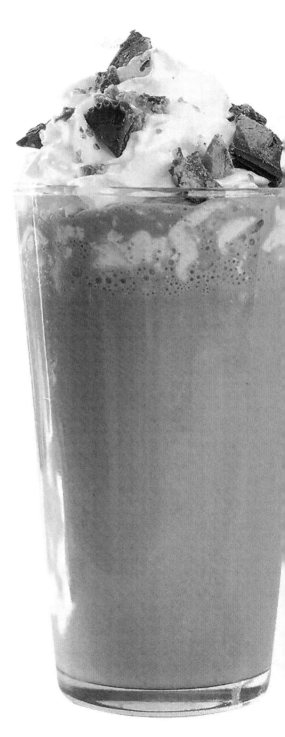

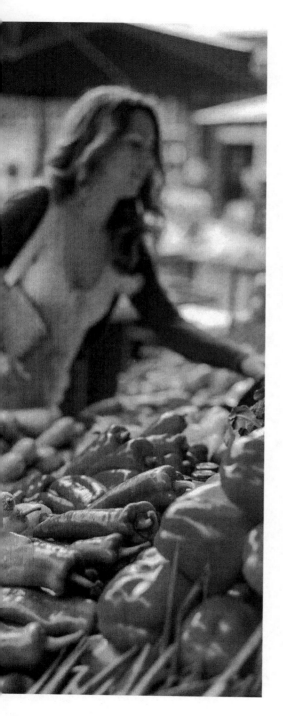

It's just a bite, right? But in fact, these "harmless nibbles" can add up to well over 300 calories a day — calories that weren't factored into your plan and that you probably don't even remember eating.

This is why the IdealPlan is built on foods you can enjoy and, most importantly, look forward to for your five daily meals. Like a chocolate peanut butter cup smoothie (included in your meal plan). And this blueprint will help you plan your snacks and cheat meals, as well.

You'll be eating foods that are going to empower you to resist junk food cravings by keeping you full and energized, and satisfying your sweet tooth, all while still meeting your calorie goal for the day. So get ready to indulge!

SECRET 3: MAXIMIZE YOUR WILLPOWER

Willpower is a limited resource, and you have to maximize it in order to be successful.

So how do you do that? One way is to fuel it by eating

frequently enough that you maintain consistent energy levels throughout the day. It comes right back to Secret #1: staying out of the hunger danger zone.

So how frequent is frequent enough? Roughly every three hours, or five times a day!

Eating five meals a day tells your brain to relax. You're getting what you need. It's about turning off the drumbeat of hunger in your head so that, when you're bombarded with unhealthy food throughout the day, you're not going to be tired and fuzzy headed, and make bad decisions.

There's a wealth of recent academic research that connects eating frequent meals with success in a fat loss program.

On the other hand, they've found that people who skip breakfast, eat a late lunch or try to cut back on meals have a VERY hard time losing weight.

By eating at regular intervals, you're giving your body and brain a steady supply of nutrients, thus stabilizing your blood sugar levels and turning off that demanding drum beat that says: 'FEED ME! FEED ME!' The result is improved mood, mental clarity and energy, there to back you up each time you make a choice about what to eat.

The second way to maximize your willpower is to conserve it by limiting the number of decisions you have to make.

Every time you make a choice about what to eat (or NOT eat), you deplete some of your willpower. Until sooner or later, you give up and find yourself sliding open the door of the soda case in the checkout line or swiping a candy bar off the rack.

By having a clear-cut meal plan, you've already made your food decisions — and you even have your treats in mind that you're looking forward to. All you have to do is stick with your plan. Avoiding decision fatigue will make your willpower undefeatable!

IDEALPLAN BREAKDOWN

You've probably experienced this firsthand, but it bears repeating: if you can't control your hunger, you can't lose weight.

That's why so many diets don't work long-term — and it's not that you failed on the diet, by the way. It's that the diet failed YOU!

The IdealPlan sets you up for success. It's designed to help you reduce your daily calories to the ideal amount for fat loss, while staying satisfied and energized with nutritious, delicious meals throughout the day.

The meal plan can be tailored based on your caloric needs and how much weight you want to lose.

WHY IT WORKS UNLIKE ANY DIET

For breakfast, you're going to have an IdealShake smoothie with the right blend of carbs and protein, and the key ingredient, Slendesta, for ultimate appetite control and fat loss.

For a snack, you'll choose an IdealBar or other snack from the list.

For lunch, you'll have another IdealShake smoothie of your choice.

For your second snack of the day, you can have your IdealBar or another snack from the list.

And for dinner, you'll whip up a simple wholesome dinner from the menu included in this book.

See, your five meals include delicious snacks and smoothies, so you'll never have to "cheat" on your diet... but it might FEEL like you are!

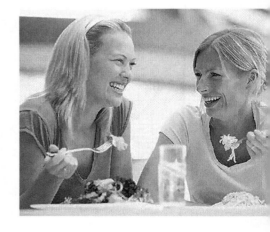

WHY FIVE MEALS A DAY?

The crux of the IdealPlan is eating a small meal approximately every three hours, which amounts to five meals a day.

It sounds counterintuitive at first, but increasing your meal frequency is fundamental to fat loss. Nutrition scientists agree that as long as we don't consume more energy (food) than we expend, dividing energy intake into more meals is ideal. That's because eating more often will help you control hunger cravings…

Have you ever come home starving after a hectic day, only to find that within minutes your healthy eating plan has completely vanished — and you're elbow-deep in a bag of chips?

If so, you're not a terrible person. In fact, you practically had no choice.

Coming back to Secret #1 and the study from Yale and University of Southern California, neuroscientists discovered that when we're hungry, we're more likely to want fatty, salty and sugary foods. To make matters worse, the part of the brain that governs self-control becomes less active.

When we DO finally eat after a long meal gap, we also tend to overestimate how much food we need to fill the void in our stomachs.

> Cravings activated
>
> Willpower deactivated
>
> + Huge plate of food
> _____
> = Disaster.

In addition to hunger management, research shows that eating more frequent meals leads to reduced insulin secretion, less insulin resistance and improved blood glucose control. All of these are beneficial to weight management and metabolism.

In a nutshell, the five-meal plan is going to help you:

Naturally decrease your calorie intake. By eating five small meals a day, you're able to avoid extreme hunger. This will make you more likely to "eat to fuel" and choose healthy foods in the portions you need.

Keep glucose and energy levels stable. Eating the right foods at regular intervals should stabilize your blood sugar levels and help you avoid the spikes that come from huge, carb heavy meals and sugary snacks. In turn, you can keep a stable level of energy to fuel your willpower and maintain a higher activity level.

Plan your meals. Increasing meal frequency actually puts you in a position to think ahead and ensure that you aren't at the mercy of fast food or convenience food. You make time to choose meals and snacks conscientiously, prepare them in advance, and have the willpower to follow through with the plan you've already made.

Feel good about yourself. One positive accomplishment leads to another! By eating approximately every three hours, you'll stay happy, satisfied and able to stick to your weight loss plan — without ever feeling deprived, hungry or fatigued.

Eating five small, but filling and nutritious meals each day is the foundation of the IdealPlan because it paves the way for certain success!

Why is This Plan 12 Weeks?

Just like having a clear-cut plan helps you stay focused, so does setting a specific timeframe for your goals. We chose 12 weeks for the IdealPlan because it's long enough to kickstart your fat loss and see noticeable results, yet not so long that it feels like what you do TODAY won't matter. Once you finish your first 12-week round, you can adjust your Plan, set new goals and start again!

SUMMARY

The IdealPlan is geared toward keeping you feeling satisfied and energized throughout the day. Remember, a diet that leaves you hungry will ALWAYS end in disaster — and let's be honest, that's pretty much every single diet out there.

"WHEN you eat is just as important as WHAT you eat"

Even if you failed to lose weight in the past with other dieting programs, with the IdealPlan you're going to learn how your nutrition habits can hinder or accelerate your results, and how following this proven system will create healthy habits for you, so you can start watching the pounds drop effortlessly.

You'll also see the three "secrets" of fat loss in action, proving that WHEN you eat is just as important as WHAT you eat.

David and I can relate to the challenge of finding a food plan that works. We're both busy parents, so we know that work, family and community obligations, along with slowing metabolism as you age, can all make fat loss seem impossible.

But with IdealPlan it is possible... and easy enough for anyone to do. Take it from our study participants who shared their experiences on page 203: this program is not based on big crazy changes, but the creation of natural lifestyle habits you can sustain longterm.

We've tested this plan with men and women who had anywhere from 20 to more than 100 pounds to lose — just to make sure it works. As you'll see for yourself, the results have been nothing short of amazing.

We can't wait to walk you through the program and help you achieve your ideal shape and ideal life. So let's get started!

Lindsey Mathews
& David Meine

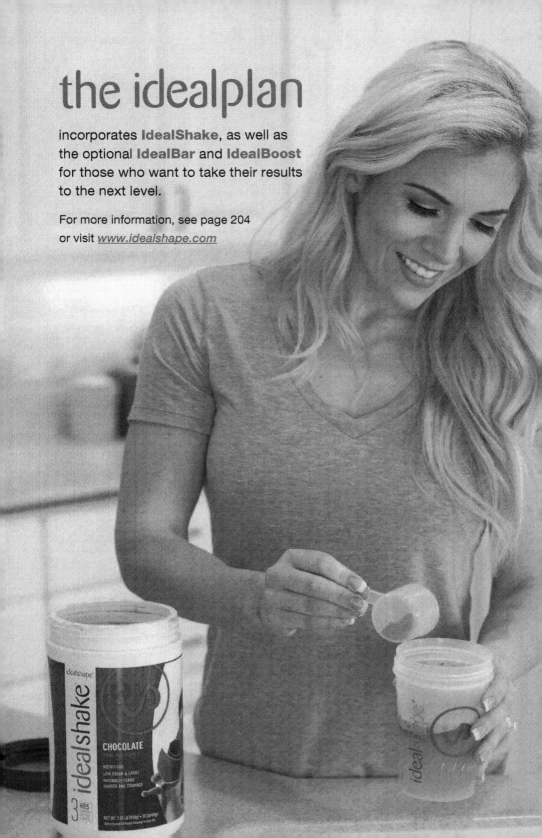

the idealplan

incorporates **IdealShake**, as well as
the optional **IdealBar** and **IdealBoost**
for those who want to take their results
to the next level.

For more information, see page 204
or visit *www.idealshape.com*

THE KEY INGREDIENT

So what's that essential ingredient in **IdealShake** we keep talking about? It's our all-natural hunger blocker called Slendesta®. This is what gives our nutrient-filled, high-quality protein smoothies a unique ability to help stimulate a feeling of fullness after a small meal. It's also in **IdealBar** and **IdealBoost** — and you won't find it in any other products on the market.

The appetite reducing process starts with something called CCK, a naturally occurring peptide in the human body released by the gut in response to food.

CCK signals to the brain that you're full and satisfied. While there is no way to just eat CCK, we've developed a special proprietary formula using protein extract from one food that triggers a high CCK release in your body: white potatoes!

Remember how we said earlier that hunger was mostly mental? Sometimes you just need to feed your body the right nutrients and retrain your brain to be satisfied with what it needs, rather than what it thinks it needs. To help start the "retraining," an appetite suppressant can do the work of telling your brain that you're full. Slendesta does just that.

Here's the most important part: Slendesta does not have the side effects of typical weight loss products. In fact, it has no known side effects at all. It's just a natural hunger blocker that's been shown to keep us full for up to three hours, right up until it's time for that next meal.

We can't say it enough: the only way to stick with your healthy meal plan and lose fat is to reduce calories without feeling tired or hungry. You can do it with the IdealPlan and your secret weapon in the fight against hunger: **Slendesta.**

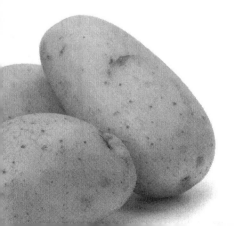

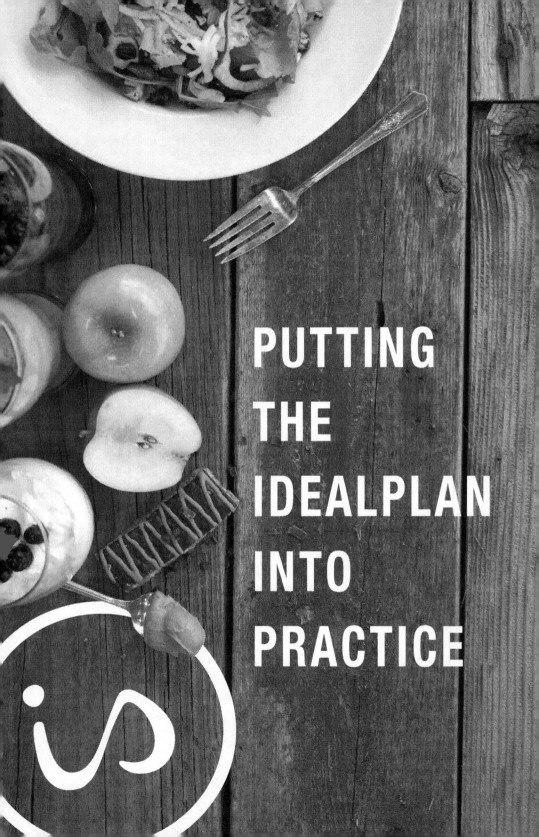

PUTTING THE IDEALPLAN INTO PRACTICE

TEN ACCELERATORS

The following fat loss accelerators are based on the three principles we shared with you in the introduction:
1) staying satisfied and energized throughout the day,
2) indulging in planned treats, and
3) maximizing your willpower by planning ahead.

As you read through this section you'll understand why we've created the IdealPlan meals in the way that we have, with these portions and these ingredients. We've put the fat loss accelerators into play throughout the IdealPlan to help you curb hunger, reduce calories, have more energy and feel prepared to make healthy choices every day.

Most of the accelerators correspond with the IdealPlan, so they're already taken care of in Phase 1! The others can be added in Phases 2 and 3 (or whenever it suits you) to reach your ideal shape even faster.

Take it at your own pace. Don't feel like you need to implement all of the "bonus" accelerators right at the start. They're grouped in order of importance, so you will see dramatic results from the beginning. More importantly, you will be building a solid foundation of nutrition habits that stick!

Phase 1 (Weeks 1-4)

1. Plan and Prep Your Meals

2. Make the Most of Breakfast

3. Include Protein in Every Meal

4. Have a Weekly Cheat Meal

5. Understand Your Macros

Phase 2 (Weeks 5-8)

6. Drink the Right Amount of Water

7. Expand Your Vegetable Repertoire

8. Reduce Your Sugar Intake

Phase 3 (Weeks 9-12)

9. Close the Kitchen at Night

10. Manage Your BLTs

Plan and Prep Your Meals

As you already know, the IdealPlan is built around five meals a day. Having a small meal approximately every three hours is a great way to fuel your body with consistent energy and keep hunger and cravings under control throughout the day.

But you might be asking yourself: How am I going to have time to prepare and eat five meals a day? I barely have time for two or three!

That's where following the IdealPlan, combined with some savvy prep tricks, comes in.

Following a meal plan is one of the simplest ways to give yourself a nutrition "makeover" without getting frazzled. No more thinking about what to eat. No more staring into the cupboard in the middle of the afternoon, starving, desperate for something to jump out at you. You have a plan in place, all your food prepped and ready to go, and you WILL be successful!

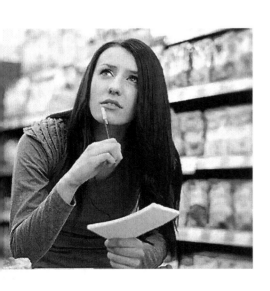

WHY IT ACCELERATES FAT LOSS

- **Keeps your calories in check.** If you're really hungry at mealtime, you're probably going to reach for the high-calorie options. However, if you have a healthy meal in mind (or even better, already prepared) you're going to grab that. Meals you prepare yourself are also usually much lower in calories, sugar and sodium than packaged foods and restaurant meals.

- **Gives your willpower a break.** Willpower is a limited resource and every time you make a choice you deplete some of it. But when you've already made a mental commitment about what to eat, you eliminate those struggles over whether to eat healthy or "cave in."

- **Saves time & money.** Eating the same things daily for a week or more ensures you use all of the food you bought and will shorten your grocery list, as well as cut down on impulse buys. If it's not on your meal plan you don't put it on your list. If it's not on your list, you don't buy it! Grocery shopping gets faster, and you can prep multiple days' worth of food at a time.

Now that you have a meal plan laid out for you, what meals or ingredients can you prepare in advance to make life easier? Here's what I do once a week on Saturdays:

For smoothies, I portion out my fruit and do any chopping and other prep work.

For dinners, I choose the IdealPlan dinner recipes I'm going to make for the coming week and cook the chicken and beef (you can do any lean meat of your choice). Then I divide them into containers and pop them into the freezer so they stay fresh. I also cook a pot of brown rice for my week's recipes.

While the rice and meat are cooking, I portion out my snacks for the next seven days into tupperware and baggies (for me, it's usually cottage cheese, beef jerky and almonds).

This is the majority of my prep for the week — done in 90 minutes!

THREE MORE WAYS TO PLAN AHEAD

Keep your shake mix and blender bottle at work or in the car, for those times when you're in a pinch.

Double or triple the IdealPlan dinner recipes so you'll have leftovers for **a few meals.**

Make all your meals the night before and put them in a freezable, insulated cooler bag that you can grab in the morning. My bag keeps food cold for 10 hours and I carry it everywhere. You can get cooler bags in big sizes, some are even as big as grocery bags!

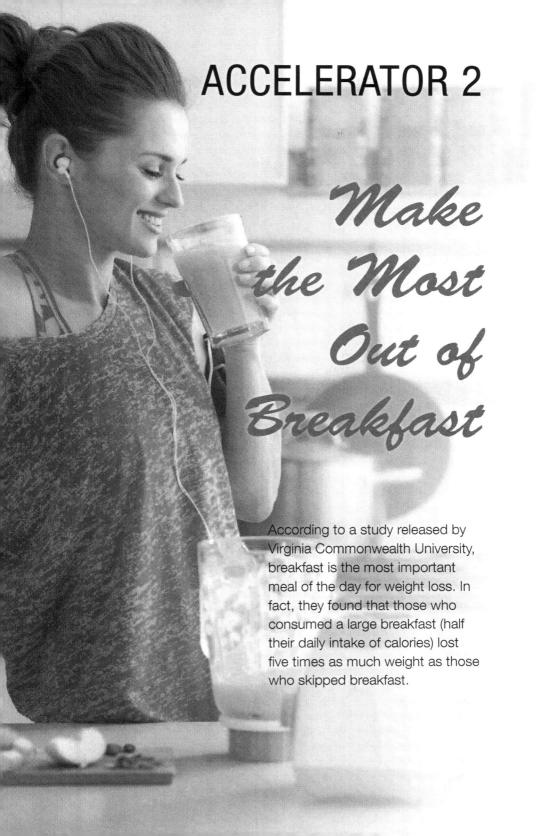

ACCELERATOR 2

Make the Most Out of Breakfast

According to a study released by Virginia Commonwealth University, breakfast is the most important meal of the day for weight loss. In fact, they found that those who consumed a large breakfast (half their daily intake of calories) lost five times as much weight as those who skipped breakfast.

Now, you don't need to consume half your calories at the crack of dawn. The IdealPlan spreads your calories out more evenly across your meals. But this study drives home an important point: eating a meal is always better than skipping a meal when it comes to losing weight. It's especially true for breakfast, which can make or break your nutrition choices for the rest of the day!

That's why the IdealPlan ensures you get a filling, low-calorie breakfast each day.

WHY IT ACCELERATES FAT LOSS

- **Provides hunger and craving control.**
  When you have a balanced meal (with proteins, carbs and fats) first thing in the morning, you'll stay full longer. It also helps with cravings later in the day by keeping your blood sugar stable. Rather than hunting for snacks in your coworker's desk, or feeling tempted to join them for fast food, when 10am or 11am rolls around you'll be calm and in control of your food choices.

- **More energy.**
  A study by the University of Kansas Medical Center shows that protein-rich breakfasts support increased physical activity and brain function. You'll feel more focused and alert after having a good breakfast. You might even start taking the stairs to work!

- **Increased fat burn with exercise.**
  If you're a morning exerciser, the right breakfast will help you get more out of your workout session. Protein will also help you increase fat burn and improve muscle tone in conjunction with a strength-

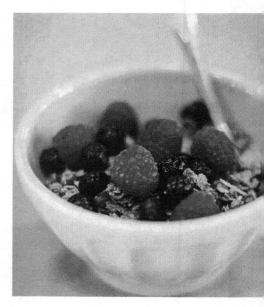

training regimen like IdealBody, by facilitating muscle repair and recovery.

The IdealPlan is all about appetite control and fueling your energy and willpower. So one of our primary goals with your meal plan was to make sure you start the day with a good breakfast That means we created your Breakfast Smoothies with a balance of carbs, proteins and fats (roughly 40/30/30). IdealShake contains a base of 11 grams of high-quality protein, and your carbs and fats come from the add-ins we suggest.

For many of us, work and school greatly dictate our eating schedules, but if you want to achieve your ideal shape, it's worth making time for breakfast! That's another reason the smoothies in the IdealPlan are great for breakfast: they're quick and convenient, so you'll never be too busy to blend one up and take it with you.

If you're not especially hungry in the morning, or you have breakfast right before a workout, a smoothie with IdealShake makes for a light and simple, yet energizing meal.

ACCELERATOR 3

Include Protein in Every Meal

If you want to achieve your fitness and fat loss goals even faster, protein is your friend! Each of your five daily meals in the IdealPlan includes protein, and that's because it's a critical macronutrient that people often don't get enough of. Having it in every meal helps ensure that you get a good amount each day.

Protein takes longer for the body to digest than carbs, so it keeps you full longer. It's also important for building muscle in conjunction with strength workouts like the ones Lindsey created for IdealBody.

Protein is made up of amino acids that are the building blocks of muscle tissue. When you lift weights, your muscles actually tear as you break them down. Protein is responsible for building them back up — and building them up even stronger than before — through a process called protein synthesis.

We know what some of you are thinking... "I don't want to look like a body builder" or "I don't want to get big." But don't underestimate the benefits of increased muscle mass!

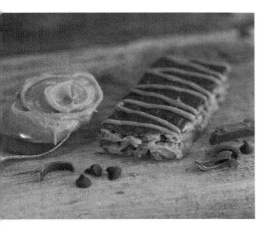

WHY IT ACCELERATES FAT LOSS

- **Increases strength and activity level.**
  With increased functional strength, daily tasks like going up stairs, bending over and lifting boxes are easier. With increased recreational strength, you can hike, ski, dance or run, no sweat. and burn lots of calories in the process!

- **Improves metabolism.**
  Our muscles are the most metabolically active tissues in our body. This means they require more calories to maintain, which in turn means our metabolism has to be faster to maintain them. The more muscle you carry, the faster your metabolism will be and the easier it will be to lose fat.

- **Puts your cheat meal to work.**
  The faster your metabolism is, the more your "cheat meal" (one of the nine accelerators) will work for you. Your body will use these weekly indulgences as fuel rather than storing them as fat.

The type of protein matters. While there might be a few grams of protein in quinoa, for example, it's still primarily a carb. Nuts and peanut butter, while they contain protein, are primarily fats. The recipes and food lists in the IdealPlan include foods we've selected as the best source of protein. IdealShake and IdealBars are also terrific protein sources and have you covered for up to three meals a day. If you are vegan or vegetarian, you can rely on beans, quinoa, lentils, nuts and soy for protein.

Some women don't want to put on a ton of muscle, but ladies, don't worry: you won't bulk up just by doing strength exercises and eating more protein. Women don't have enough testosterone to build the kind of muscle mass that would make you look too big or like a bodybuilder. However, you will get a shapelier physique. You've seen the skinny person who still looks somewhat flabby, right? When you build muscle mass, you won't bulk up but you WILL enhance your body shape and create firmer skin. So bring on the sleek curves!

Have a Weekly Cheat Meal

Cheaters do prosper! Having a cheat meal will help you stick with your healthy eating plan. If you were worried about surviving a fat loss plan without your favorite foods, you can breathe a sigh of relief!

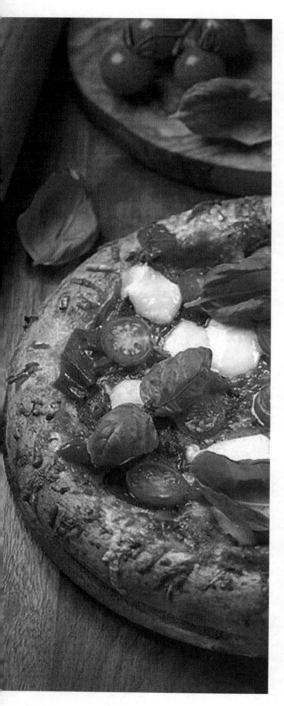

And if you're worried about going "off the rails" after the first bite of each indulgence, don't be. We'll be giving you three strategies for enjoying your cheat meal guilt-free, then jumping right back on track with your nutrition goals.

WHY IT ACCELERATES FAT LOSS:

- **Fits with your social life.**
  No one wants to be a hermit! Having a weekly cheat meal lets you enjoy date nights, barbecues, holidays and birthday parties.

- **Boosts your willpower.**
  Staying true to your nutrition plan all week isn't always easy, but passing up your favorite foods is made easier when you know you can have them for your weekly cheat meal.

- **Has a hormonal benefit.**
  Prolonged dieting can really decrease your leptin stores, which makes it hard to continue to lose fat. Leptin regulates the amount of fat stored in our bodies by adjusting our feelings of hunger. If our leptin levels go

down we'll feel hungrier and have more cravings. One way to keep leptin levels as high as possible is to splurge on a good, higher calorie meal once a week.

Each week, look at your meal plan and decide when you want to have your cheat meal and what you want to indulge in. Don't forget to choose a strategy, one from below or one of your own, to get right back on track after the meal.

The best way to make your cheat meal truly guilt-free is to keep it from creeping out into other meals, snacks and bites.

TRIED AND TRUSTED STRATEGIES

- **Give your cheat meal a start and end time.**
  If you start dinner at 6pm and plan on having dessert around 7pm, your end time might be 7:15 or 7:30. This will prevent your cheat meal from spilling into later meals or BLTs (see the accelerator about "bites, licks and tastes").

- **Set a plate limit.**
  For holidays and potlucks, a start and end time might feel like you're giving yourself free reign to binge for two hours. If you're worried about this, give yourself a plate limit instead — say, one plate for dinner and one for dessert.

- **Restaurant meals are great "cheats."**
  Rather than standing around the buffet for hours or sitting in your kitchen staring at a half-eaten gallon of ice cream, at a restaurant you order your meal, eat it and you're finished.

What should you have for your cheat meal? The beauty of this is that you can really have anything you want... but not everything you want. Instead of feeling like you have to count your cheat meal calories, just have "moderate" portions - say, one serving of pizza and one serving of pie, instead of 3-4 servings.

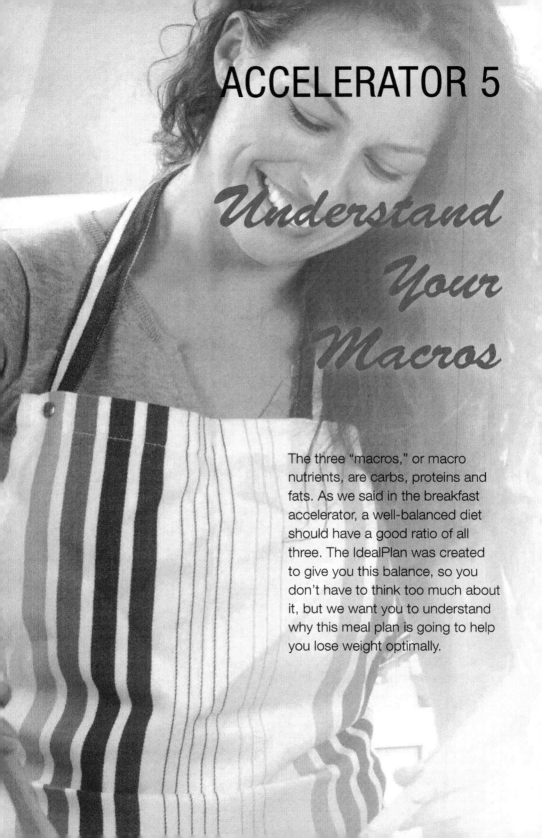

ACCELERATOR 5

Understand Your Macros

The three "macros," or macro nutrients, are carbs, proteins and fats. As we said in the breakfast accelerator, a well-balanced diet should have a good ratio of all three. The IdealPlan was created to give you this balance, so you don't have to think too much about it, but we want you to understand why this meal plan is going to help you lose weight optimally.

WHY IT ACCELERATES FAT LOSS

- If your diet is too low in carbs, you'll feel very low in energy, which can affect your physical activity level. You could eventually suffer from a slow metabolism.

- If your diet is too low in protein, you could lose muscle, which can result in a slower metabolism and flabbiness rather than a lean looking body.

- If your diet is too low in fat you could suffer from hormonal imbalances and you'll probably be really hungry. Sometimes we make an enemy out of fat, but it's important to get enough fats in your diet.

- The body process each macronutrient at a different rate, so a balance helps satisfy your hunger longer, as you'll see in the following Guide to Macronutrients.

So what's a good balance? The ratio that is usually a good starting point, and that IdealPlan is built around, is approximately 40/30/30. This means roughly 40% of your calories come from carbs, 30% from protein and 30% from fat. Notice I said percent of your calories, not percent of your portions.

Here's an example. Let's say you're a 200-lb woman on a 1,800 calorie plan. Your breakdown would look like this:

Carbs: 40% of 1,800 calories is 720 calories. Each gram of carbs has 4 calories. Divide 720 calories by 4 and you have 180g carbs.

Protein: 30% of 1,800 calories is 540 calories. Each gram of protein has 4 calories. Divide 540 calories by 4 and you have 135g protein.

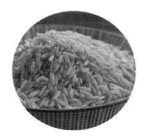
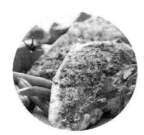
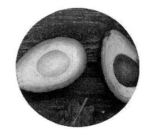

Fat: 30% of 1,800 calories is 540 calories. Each gram of fat has 9 calories (you'll see that's quite a bit more than the calories in protein and carbs). Divide 540 calories by 9 and you have 60g fat.

So our 200-lb example woman should have 180g carbs, 135g protein and 60g fat. Sometimes this is more math than people want to think about, and that's why we've done it for you in the meal plan.

A GUIDE TO MACRONUTRIENTS

CARBS

Carbs are your body's preferred and most efficient source of energy, very important in fueling exercise.

Simple Carbs:

- Made up of simple sugars

- Broken up and absorbed quickly by the body

- Can more dramatically affect blood sugar levels

- Most simple carbs (with the exception of fruit, honey, etc.) should be avoided most times

of the day, but can actually be beneficial during the pre and post workout meals.

Examples: fruit, honey, soda, candy, cakes, snack foods, white bread products

Complex Carbs:

- Take longer to digest and absorb

- Help stabilize blood sugar levels and avoid spikes

- Contain important vitamins and minerals

Examples: vegetables, whole grains, brown rice, sweet potatoes

FATS

Fats are an essential nutrient, another source of energy and they slow digestion so they help us feel full longer.

Good Fats:

- Boost heart health, lower cholesterol, boosts skin, hair and cellular health, lower blood pressure, help prevent blood clots and strokes, boosts hormone production

- Monounsaturated, polyunsaturated, even some saturated fats such as coconut and coconut oil Examples: Avocado, nuts, nut butter, seeds, olive oil, fatty fish, flax

Bad Fats:

- Man-made through a process called hydrogenation

- Increase "bad" cholesterol and lower "good" cholesterol, increase insulin levels, and possibly lead to diabetes

- Look for the words "partially hydrogenated" on the ingredient list and if you see it, avoid it at all costs!

Examples: You'll find them in most snack foods, chips, margarine, cookies, fried foods, and even some seemingly healthy foods such as crackers, some salad dressings and some "healthy" cereals.

Proteins

Protein is made up of amino acids that are the building blocks of muscle tissue. Protein synthesis (the process of building new muscle tissue) is optimal when you eat protein at regular intervals throughout the day. That's why it's included in each of your five meals.

Here are some examples of good protein sources:

- Breakfast and Lunch: IdealShake, Greek yogurt

- Snacks: IdealBar, beef jerky, cottage cheese, string cheese and turkey slices, tuna packet, hard boiled egg

- Dinner: Chicken, turkey sausage, beef, any lean meat

Note for vegans and vegetarians: While beans, quinoa and lentils are primarily a carb source, they do have protein in them. And while nuts and nut butter are primarily a fat source, they also contain protein. There are also vegan protein powders available. So don't worry, it is possible to get plenty of protein in your diet as a vegan or vegetarian!

Drink the Right Amount of Water

Dehydration will wreck your fitness goals faster than you can say "I'll have an iced tea." Water is a natural appetite suppressant, improves metabolic function and helps you exercise with more intensity, so it's one of your best weapons in weight loss!

WHY IT ACCELERATES FAT LOSS

Improves metabolic function.
Our bodies are primarily made up of water. Even just slight dehydration can cause muscle aches, grumpiness, dizziness, lethargy, mental fatigue, poor digestion and irregularity. When we don't drink enough water, toxins in the body don't get flushed out, which essentially impairs the body's ability to balance blood sugar and metabolize cholesterol... opening the door to diabetes and obesity.

Suppresses appetite naturally.
When we feel hungry, sometimes we're actually just thirsty. Try drinking a big glass of water and waiting 15-20 minutes to see if you're still hungry. If you're legitimately hungry but it's not time for your next meal, drink a big glass of water (or IdealBoost) and it will help tide you over until your next meal.

Fuels your workouts.
Exercise energy doesn't just come from food! Not drinking enough water causes our bodies to be tired and sluggish. On the other hand, starting your workout well hydrated will enable you to work out at a higher intensity.

Cuts down your less healthy beverages.
Thanks to clever advertising and bottle labeling tricks, sometimes we unconsciously turn to soda and juice to quench our thirst. when all we wanted was a refreshing glass of H20.

How much water do you really need? We recommend that you drink anywhere from 12-16 cups of water per day (one cup is 8 ounces). Definitely NO LESS than 10 cups per day. And if your goal is weight loss, drink on the higher end, including having two cups of water about 30 minutes before your meals.

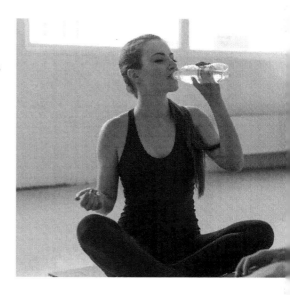

If you're drinking much less than this, it's good to build up to your ideal water intake slowly. Start by counting your cups of water on your first day. On your second day, try to add two cups, and on your third day add two more and so on until you reach 12-16 cups.

YOUR HYDRATION STRATEGY

You're probably thinking "How on earth do I drink that much?" There are two ways to make sure you get enough water each day and it really depends on your personality. If you're a schedule oriented person, try this: drink two cups immediately upon waking, then two more by 9am, four cups by noon, four more cups by 3pm, and four more by 6pm.

Some of you may prefer to just sip on your gallon throughout the day and that's fine too. Either way, try to get at least half of your water in by midday to make sure you're keeping on top of it (and so you won't be up all night in the bathroom).

You'll also be following each IdealShake smoothie with 8 oz of water to activate the hunger-blocking ingredient. This will count as one of your cups!

Note: When you increase your water intake you need to make sure your electrolytes stay balanced, which may require you to increase your sodium intake. If you increase your water slowly, you should feel just fine. But if you increase it quickly you might notice that you start to feel slight headaches; to bring your electrolytes back into balance, just add a little more salt to your food!

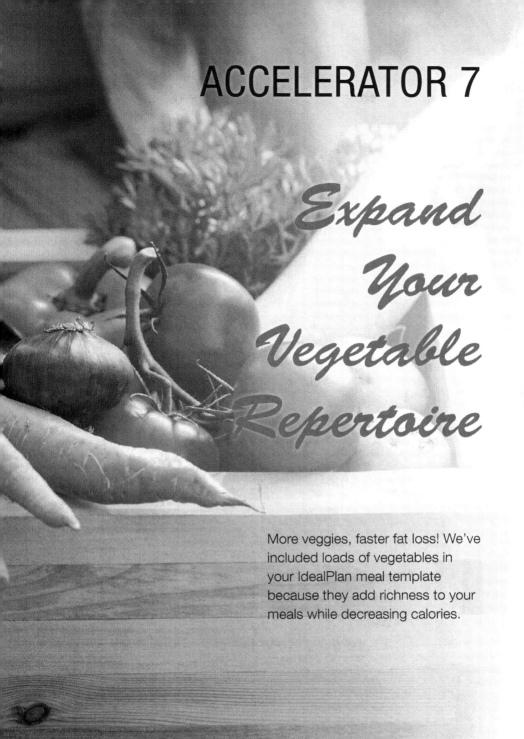

Expand Your Vegetable Repertoire

More veggies, faster fat loss! We've included loads of vegetables in your IdealPlan meal template because they add richness to your meals while decreasing calories.

WHY IT ACCELERATES FAT LOSS

Lowers calories.
Most veggies are low in calories and high in fiber, so you can snack on them anytime without having to "count" or factor the calories into your meal plan.*

Boosts health.
Vegetables may reduce the risk of heart disease, obesity and Type 2 diabetes, and may protect against certain cancers, as well as help you maintain a healthy blood pressure. Veggies are a good source of vitamin A, C, folic acid and potassium.

Provides appetite control.
Because they're high in fiber and water, vegetables are natural appetite suppressants. With a bigger helping of veggies on your plate, you'll feel full despite smaller portions of the high-calorie stuff.

A TIP ON TRYING NEW VEGGIES

If you're feeling adventurous, you can begin to incorporate new vegetables into your meal plan or new ways of preparing them. We've found some of our favorites by just trying out new ones that we've never heard of, like jicama, lemon cucumber, okra and chayote.

When you want to try a new veggie, try preparing it three ways:

- Slice it and try it raw with some salt.

- Dice it up and steam it.

- Roast it.

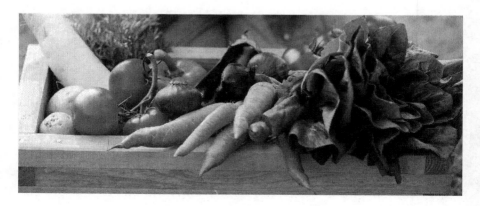

Most veggies are really good in at least one of these ways!

GREEN SMOOTHIES

Are you on the green smoothie train yet? You can get a lot of servings of vegetables this way! The Tropical Greens and Peachy Greens smoothies in the IdealPlan are a good start, especially if you like your smoothies a little sweeter. To go fully green, try replacing some of your Breakfast or Lunch Smoothies with your own green mix — add spinach, kale, carrots, cucumber, bell pepper, tomato, or whatever you feel like. Vegetables blend well with water or almond milk, some fruit and a scoop of Vanilla IdealShake!

* Most vegetables are low in calories and high in fiber, so they'll fill you up before you can overdo it. That's why we give you the green light to load up on these and add as many as you like to your IdealPlan meals. However, not all veggies are "freebies": potatoes, carrots, squash, corn and peas are starchy carbs that could hinder your fat loss, if you eat too much of them. For these vegetables, you'll want to stick with the portions in your meal plan.

ACCELERATOR 8

Reduce Your Sugar Intake

One of the biggest fears people have when starting a diet is that they'll have to give up sweets. It's no secret that Americans are addicted to sugar. It's almost impossible to avoid it, because it's added to most of our food, creating a dependence that is hard to escape from!

Overcoming a "sweet tooth" is essential to fat loss, though. In fact, if you're overweight, there is a pretty good chance that you've had too much sugar in your diet.

Here's the good news: there is a way to change your appetite for sugar, and the IdealPlan is going to help you do it.

WHY IT ACCELERATES FAT LOSS

Lowers calories.
Rarely do we have just a taste of something sugary. Since we don't feel full after eating foods filled with refined sugar, we keep eating and eating, seeking to trigger those "feel good" chemicals in the brain. Processed foods that are high in sugar are usually high in calories, so avoiding the slippery sugar slope will save you hundreds of calories a day.

Reduces energy spikes and dips.
Sugary foods usually lead to a spike in blood sugar, followed by a crash. It's especially true if they don't contain fiber and other ingredients that take longer for the body to process, such as complex carbs or protein. Kick these sugar crashes and you'll have more sustained energy throughout the day, which will keep your willpower strong.

Boosts health and prevents disease.
Excessive sugar consumption is one of the biggest causes of type 2 diabetes, as well as many other chronic conditions. It can also impair your body's ability to fight off colds and flus. A strong immune system is essential to achieving your ideal shape and keeping it.

Cutting back on sugar can be a challenge, and that's why we've made it a Phase 2 accelerator. One of the keys to successful fat loss is not attempting to make too many changes at once. Thankfully, because you're following the plan, your sugar intake is already going to be much lower.

Chances are you're still going to face temptations — but the IdealPlan will help you conquer them. It comes back to the three secrets of fat loss that create the foundation of the plan:

1. **Controlling hunger and cravings.**
   Hunger is mostly mental, and when you're craving sugary foods, it's often a result of hunger that then triggers those cravings in your brain. By managing your hunger, the IdealPlan is going to reduce these cravings.

2. **Indulging in treats.**
   Cold turkey? It never worked for me. A more effective way to reduce sugar consumption, without the boomerang effect, is by replacing unhealthy treats with healthy ones. Instead of a candy bar or cookie, you can have a S'mores or Strawberry Yogurt IdealBar. Fruit and fruit smoothies will also satisfy your sweet tooth while giving you plenty of fiber and vitamins and minerals.

3. **Fueling your willpower.**
   Minimizing choices with a clear-cut plan, and planning your treats, will put less strain on your willpower. You've already made up your mind. Since you know you're going to have berries for your snack or a decadent dessert for your weekly cheat meal, it's easier to say "no" to the donuts, muffins, etc. that crop up that aren't part of your plan.

DON'T DRINK YOUR SUGAR!

As you reduce your sugar intake, your body is going to try to get its sugar fix in sneaky ways! In Phase 2, you'll have to pay close attention to your beverage choices. Juices, sodas, iced teas and many other drinks are packed with sugar. Yes, even juice: the more fiber that accompanies carbohydrates, the less of an adverse physiological response the sugar will have, and fiber is largely eliminated from juice.

Here are a few ways to avoid "drinking your sugar" while following the IdealPlan:

- Drinking more water (another Phase 2 fat loss accelerator) should help diminish your hankering for other beverages — if only because you don't want to spend the whole day in the bathroom!

- For an energy boost, replace sodas and energy drinks with a flavorful glass of IdealBoost,

which has 0g of sugar. It
contains green tea and caffeine
(both improve metabolism,
a bonus!) and our signature
hunger blocker, Slendesta.

- If you're a coffee lover, trade a
  frozen latte for a blended Salted
  Caramel Latte smoothie or a
  Minty Mocha smoothie from the
  plan. It's less sugar, plus you're
  getting protein and hun-ger-
  blocking benefits.

If you can hold out, your cravings
will start to lose their intensity and
you'll enjoy the taste of lower sugar
foods. Our guess is that by Phase
3, you won't even crave sugary
foods!

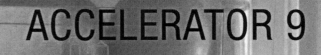

Close the Kitchen at Night

We recommend "closing the kitchen" three hours before bedtime. There's some controversy around this idea, so before we go any further, we'll say this: current research has shown that as long as you're eating the right food in the right amounts, it technically doesn't matter when you eat it. The calories you eat after 8pm won't magically "turn to fat."

But there's a different reason that closing the kitchen at night is important for fat loss. It has to do with typical behavior patterns...

Just think back to the last time you went into the kitchen at night while watching your favorite TV show. You were only going to have a taste of peanut butter — it's healthy, right? So you had your bite, and then you saw the bag of chocolate chips and decided to just have a couple. Then maybe you wanted a little of the peanut butter and chocolate chips together. So you got out your spoon and started dipping. Next thing you knew, you'd eaten a lot more than you meant to.

It's an endless cycle!

If you're following the IdealPlan and eating five meals per day, you've probably already had all of your calories by the time evening rolls around. Like you'll see with the accelerator about managing "BLTs" (that stands for "bites, licks and tastes"), unplanned calories are exactly what you want to avoid!

CHOOSING YOUR CUTOFF TIME

Planned cheat meals are great, fun and satisfying, but unplanned cheat meals can leave you feeling guilty — a feeling that often leads to a downward spiral. Creating your own "kitchen closed"rule will help you stay focused. We recommend not even GOING into the kitchen after cutoff time so you won't be tempted.

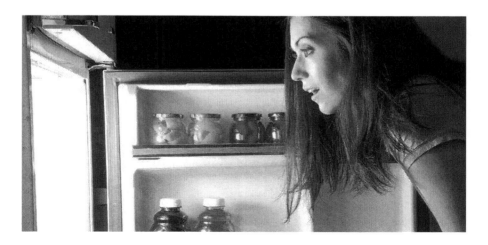

So when should your kitchen cutoff time be? This is up to you and when you feel the most tempted, but a good starting point is three hours before bedtime. If you go to bed at 11pm, have a "no eating after 8pm" rule. When dinner is done, clean the kitchen. If you have a snack a little later or if your kids do, clean up after that and then turn off the light. If the kitchen is clean and the light is off, it helps you to stay out!

Exception to the Rule:
Some people like to have dessert or a snack around 8pm, and we have lots of people who choose to have an IdealShake around that time because it's "like dessert."

As long as your evening snack is part of your five-meal plan and included in your daily calorie goal, it's no problem.

See the FAQ for guidance on how to factor a dessert IdealShake smoothie into your meal plan!

ACCELERATOR 10

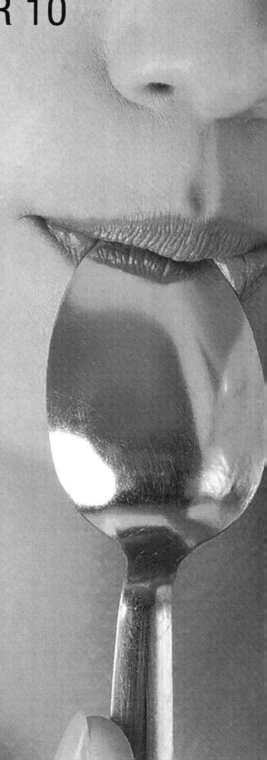

Manage Your B.L.T.s

By this point you've heard us talk about "BLTs" a few times. It's not a bacon, lettuce and tomato sandwich — it stands for *Bites, Licks and Tastes*. It refers to eating a little of anything that isn't part of your meal plan.

A Cornell University study found that most people wouldn't have a clue if we ate an extra 300 calories in a day. The study author, Brian Wansink, said in his bestselling book Mindless Eating that people who are overweight tend to underestimate calories by 30-40%!

If you've hit a fat loss plateau, BLTs could easily be the culprit. We've seen them add up to 300 calories a day or more in people's diets.

Here's an example:

A few bites of cereal out of the bag as you pass by
= 40 calories

2 Hershey kisses from the jar on your coworker's desk
= 50 calories

Licking peanut butter off the knife when you make your kids' lunch
= 35 calories

Bites of dinner as you make it
= 75 calories

The rest of your kids' dinner that you just can't bear to throw away
= 75 calories

An after dinner candy because you have to end with something sweet
= 25 calories

That's up to 300 calories in a day! That adds up to 2,100 extra calories over the course of a week, which is almost a full pound (3,500 extra calories = 1 pound). So this is either weight gain, or fat you could be losing that you AREN'T.

TIPS FOR AVOIDING BLT'S

BLTs aren't easy to avoid, but even just being aware of the habit will help you start to curb calories. Here are some strategies that might help you limit BLTs:

- Tie a ribbon around your wrist or finger that reminds you whenever you look down at your hand not to have BLTs.

- Keep paper towels on the counter in arm's reach so you can quickly wipe food off the spoons and knives you're cooking with so you aren't tempted to lick!

- Use Post-Its and post your goals and even the words "NO BLTS" everywhere you look.

- Make a sign above the sink that says "WASH ME" reminding you to hurry and rinse off your dishes and utensils before licking them clean!

Now, avoiding BLTs isn't the same as choosing to have a sliver of cake to satisfy a craving, instead of having a whole piece. Sometimes that's exactly the right thing to do. We're talking about the tendency to peck at food throughout the day... and even just being aware of the habit will help you start to curb calories. If there's a certain temptation you just can't resist, see if you can find a way to include it in your meal plan or have it for your cheat meal.

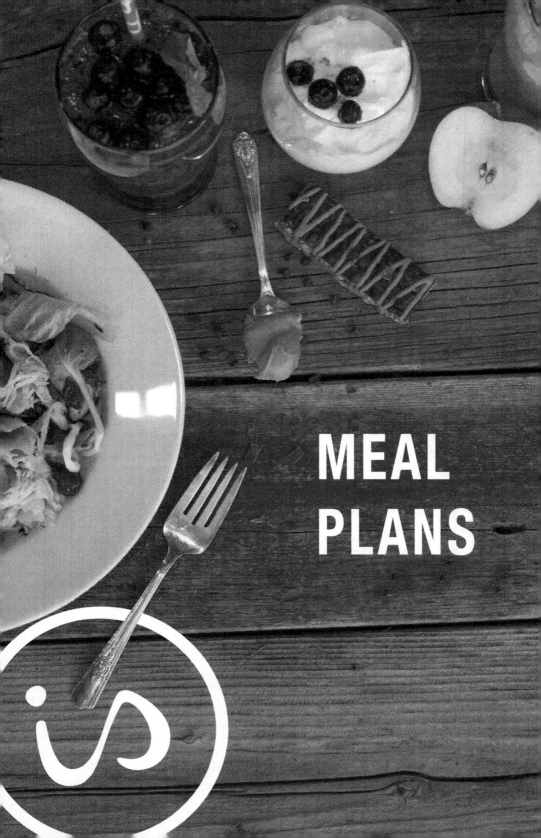

MEAL
PLANS

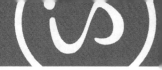
WOMEN UNDER 140 lbs

If you're a woman currently weighing under 140 lbs, here is everything you need to put IdealPlan into action today! This meal plan is targeted to your gender and body weight range to help you reach your goals faster.

Remember: Make sure to use the recipes and food lists that go with your specific meal plan. The calorie amounts and portions of each macronutrient (carbs, proteins and fats) are slightly different for each weight/gender category.

This program is simple on purpose: we've done all the math for you, giving you the calorie amount and balance of carbs, proteins and fats that are generally ideal for fat loss for your weight range. We've also selected foods that fit great with this template, but if you prefer to use your own comparable substitutions, that's fine too!

Because everybody is different and physical activity levels vary from person to person, you can use the check-in points at the end of Phase 1 and Phase 2 (see FAQ) to adjust the plan according to your results.

Bookmark the next 4 pages for daily reference!

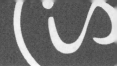

Five-Meal Template

Breakfast Smoothie

1 scoop IdealShake

1 large serving fruit (see fruit list)

1 c. any milk (see milk list)

Or: choose from the recipes that follow

Mid-Morning Snack

1 IdealBar

Or: 1 Protein A List Option

1 Carb B List Option

Lunch Smoothie

1 scoop IdealShake

1 Carb A List serving

1 Fat A List serving

1 c. any milk

Or: choose from the recipes that follow

Mid-Afternoon Snack

1 Protein A List Option

1 Carb B List Option

Or: choose from the recipes that follow

Optional: 1 IdealBoost stick pack

Dinner

1 serving any lean meat (3-4 oz - approx size of your palm)

1 Fat B serving

Unlimited vegetables*

Or: choose from the recipes that follow

Approximate daily calories: **1200**

40% carbs | 30% proteins | 30% fats

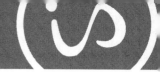

Food Lists

Milk Options

Almond Milk

Soy Milk

Skim Milk

Low fat Milk

Unsweetened Coconut Milk

Coconut Water

Rice Milk

Fruit Servings

1 banana

1 apple

1 orange

1 peach

1 pear

1 mango

1 tangerines

2 apricots

2 kiwis

1 c. berries/cherries/pineapple

1 ½ c. any melon (watermelon, cantaloupe, honeydew, etc.)

1 ½ c. grapes

1 c. any fruit juice/veggie juice

Or: Any fruit for approx 100 calories

Carb A Options (Shake Add-Ins)

¼ c. oats

1 T. chia seeds

½ fruit serving (see fruit list)

2 T. PB2 peanut butter powder

1 T. Honey/Agave/Real Maple Syrup

¼ c. Plain Cheerios (stirred in)

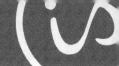

1 light yogurt

1 low fat graham cracker

Or: Any low fat carb for approx 75 calories

Carb B List (Small Snacks)

1 flavored rice cake

½ c. low sugar cereal (Plain Cheerios, Rice Chex, Wheaties, etc)

1 low fat graham cracker

½ serving whole wheat crackers

½ serving pop chips/baked chips

½ serving fruit (see fruit list)

Or: Any low fat carb for approx 50 calories

Protein A Servings (Shake Add-Ins/Snack Options)

½ c. low fat cottage cheese

¾ c. fat free plain Greek yogurt

½ scoop whey protein

1 80-100 calorie flavored Greek yogurt (e.g., Dannon Light n Fit Greek)

¾ c. liquid egg whites (can be added to shakes to make it smooth and creamy)

1 egg (hard boiled is easily transportable)

1 oz beef jerky

3 oz turkey slices

1 low fat string cheese

1 serving tuna

Or: Any protein for approx 100 calories

Fat A Serving (Shake Add-Ins)

1 T. peanut butter

½ avocado

1 T. flax seed

1 T. coconut oil

1 T. coconut flakes

½ oz dark chocolate

Or: Any low sugar fat for approx 100 calories

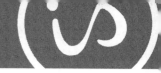
Fat B List (Dinner Options)

1 oz cheese

1 T. any nuts/seeds/nut butter

1 c. feta cheese

1 T. any oil (coconut, extra virgin olive oil, grapeseed oil, etc)

1 T. any salad dressing

½ avocado

Or: Any low sugar fat for approx 100 calories

Freebie Shake Add-Ins

1 T. Sugar free, fat free pudding powder

1 T. cocoa powder

Any Extracts - vanilla, coconut, almond, maple, orange, etc Sugar Free
Syrups (e.g., Torani and DaVinci)

¼ t. Crystal Light mix

Any vegetables*

*Vegetable Cheat Sheet

Fibrous veggies are allowed with any meal in any amount (e.g., asparagus, broccoli, Brussels sprouts, cabbage, cauliflower, celery, okra, cucumber, eggplant, collard greens, tomato, leek, lettuce, any mushroom, green onion, onion, bell pepper, radish, snow peas, spinach, zucchini, fennel, green beans, pickles).

Carrots, peas and squash are not "free" veggies but can be enjoyed occasionally.

Corn and potatoes are counted as grains/carbs in the meal plan.

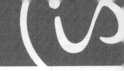
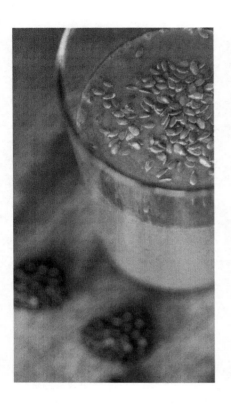

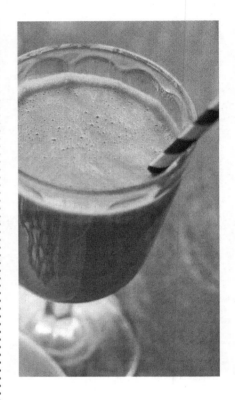

Black Berry Boost

1 scoop Vanilla IdealShake

1 c. unsweetened almond milk

1 c. fresh blackberries

Ice cubes

Chocolate Banana

1 scoop Chocolate IdealShake

1 c. unsweetened almond milk

1 banana

Ice cubes

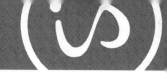

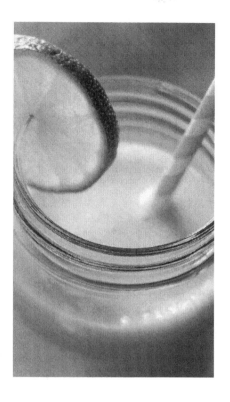

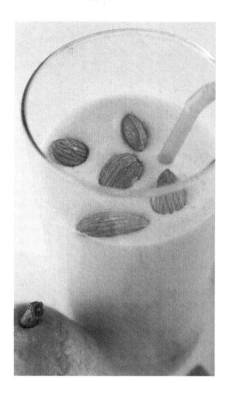

Key Lime Pie

1 scoop Vanilla IdealShake

1 c. unsweetened almond milk

1 T. lime juice

1 low fat graham cracker*

Ice cubes

Graham cracker subs for the fruit in your breakfast shake

Almond Pear Spice

1 scoop Vanilla IdealShake

1 c. unsweetened almond milk

½ banana

½ pear

1 t. cinnamon

1 t. almond extract

Ice cubes

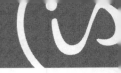

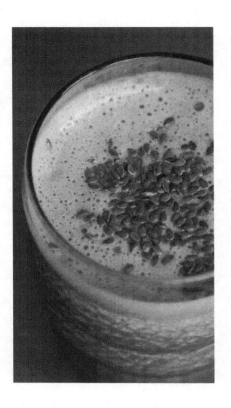

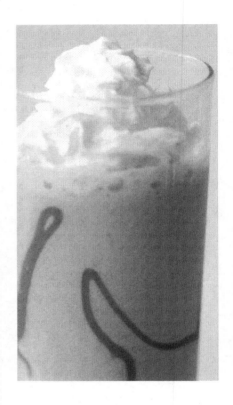

Tropical Greens

1 scoop Vanilla IdealShake

1 c. coconut water

½ c. strawberries

½ c. pineapple

1 c. spinach

Ice cubes

Salted Caramel Pumpkin Latte

1 scoop Mocha or Vanilla IdealShake

½ c. coffee, cooled

½ c. unswt almond milk

2 T. canned pumpkin

½ banana

1-2 T. sugar free Torani Salted
    Caramel Syrup

Pinch of sea salt

Ice cubes

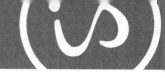

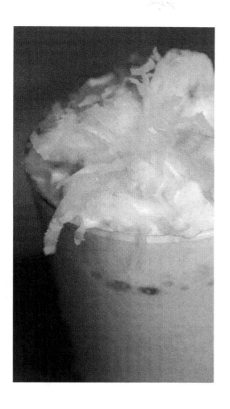

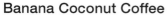

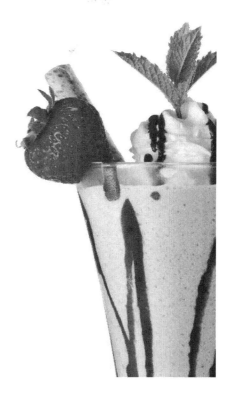

Banana Coconut Coffee

1 scoop Mocha IdealShake

1 c. unswt coconut milk

1 banana

1-2 T. sugar free Torani Coconut Syrup

Ice cubes

Triple Chocolate Berry

1 scoop Chocolate or Strawberry
   IdealShake

1 c. Hood Carb Countdown Chocolate
   Milk

¾ c. frozen strawberries

1 T. sugar free chocolate pudding
   powder

Ice cubes

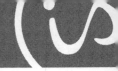

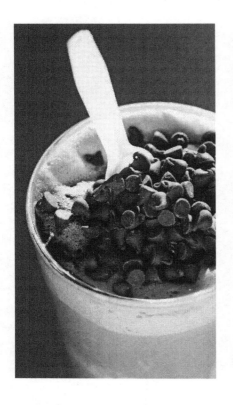

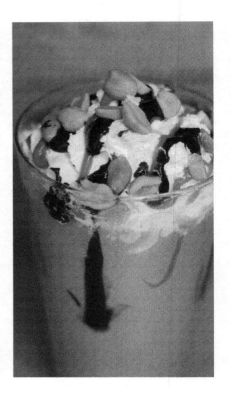

Minty Mocha

1 scoop Mocha IdealShake

1 c. unsweetened almond milk or
    cooled coffee

½ t. peppermint extract

Ice cubes

Have one piece of fruit on the side.

Candybar

1 scoop Chocolate IdealShake

1 c. unsweetened almond milk

2 T. PB2 peanut butter powder (in
    place of fruit in template)

1 t. cocoa powder

2 t. sugar free caramel syrup

Ice cubes

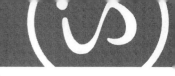

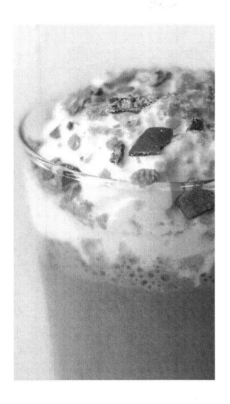

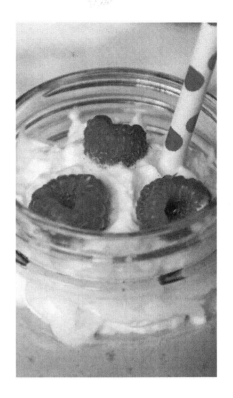

The Butter-Finger

1 scoop Chocolate IdealShake

1 c. Hood Carb Countdown Chocolate milk

1 T. peanut butter

1 T. sugar free fat free butterscotch pudding powder

¼ c. oats

½ T. unsweetened cocoa

Sweetener to taste

Ice cubes

Raspberry Cheesecake

1 scoop Vanilla IdealShake

1 c. unsweetened almond milk

½ c. frozen/fresh raspberries

1 graham cracker square

½ oz dark chocolate*

1 T. cottage cheese

Ice cubes

Dark chocolate can be sprinkled over the top or blended in

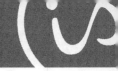

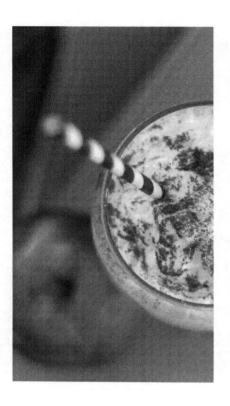

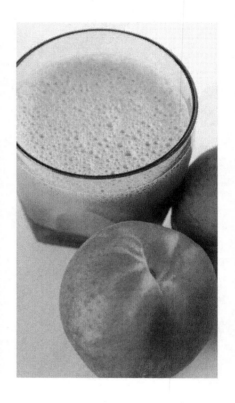

Apple Pie A La Mode

1 scoop Vanilla IdealShake

1 c. unsweetened almond milk

¼ c. unsweetened applesauce

2 T. vanilla Greek yogurt

½ t. apple pie spice

1 T. oats*

1 T. peanut butter

Ice cubes

Sprinkle the oats over the top of the shake

Peachy Greens

1 scoop Vanilla IdealShake

½ c. water

½ c. orange juice

½ peach, pitted

½ avocado

1 c. spinach

Ice cubes

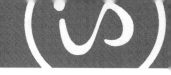

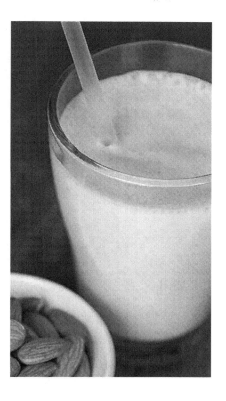

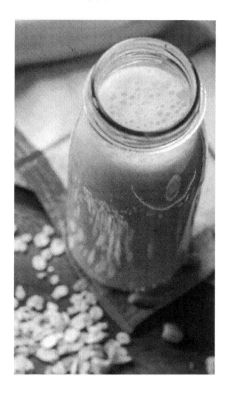

Honey Nut

1 scoop Vanilla IdealShake

1 c. unsweetened almond milk

2 T. PB2 peanut butter powder

1 t. honey

1 T. almond butter

Ice cubes

Peanut Butter Cookie

1 scoop Chocolate or Vanilla
  IdealShake

1 c. unsweetened almond milk

¼ c. oats

1 T. peanut butter

Ice cubes

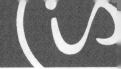

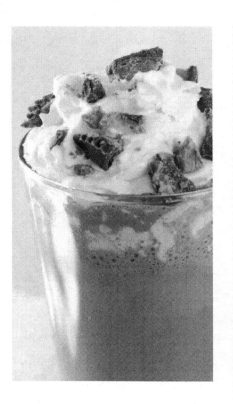

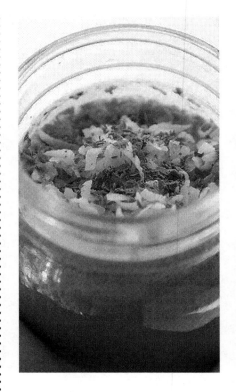

Chocolate Peanut Butter Cup

1 scoop Chocolate IdealShake

1 c. unsweetened almond milk

2 T. PB2 peanut butter powder

1 T. Peanut butter

Ice cubes

Almond Delight

1 scoop Chocolate IdealShake

1 c. dark chocolate almond milk

¼ c. oats

¼ c. part skim ricotta

1 T. coconut flakes

Ice cubes

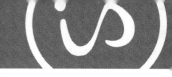

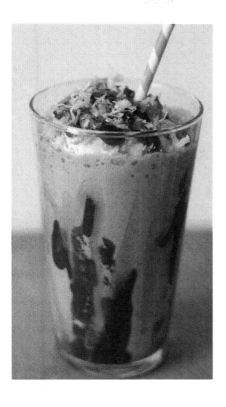

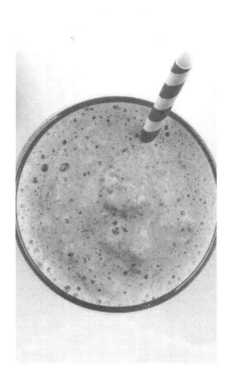

Caramel Coconut Cookie

1 scoop Chocolate IdealShake

1 c. unswt coconut milk

¼ T. coconut extract

1 T. sugar free caramel syrup ice cream topping

1 T. sugar free chocolate syrup ice cream topping

1 T. coconut oil, melted*

Ice cubes

Melt the coconut oil and then drizzle slowly into shake while blender is mixing to prevent clumping.

Berries n Cream

1 scoop Strawberry IdealShake

1 c. unswt almond milk

⅓ c. frozen raspberries

⅓ c. frozen strawberries

1 T. sugar free french vanilla creamer

1 T. fat free sugar free vanilla pudding mix

2 T. flax seeds

Ice cubes

67

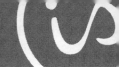

Optional:

1 IdealBoost Stick Pack drink on the side with your snack!

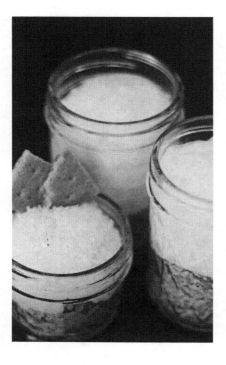

Coconut Cream Pie

1 container Coconut Dannon Light n Fit Greek yogurt

1 low fat graham cracker, crumbled

Stir graham cracker crumbs into yogurt

Tuna "Sandwich"

1 oz tuna

½ T. light mayo

1 lightly salted rice cake

Mix tuna and mayo and spread over the rice cake

Fruit and Eggs

¾ c. grapes

1 hardboiled egg

Turkey Sandwich

1 slice low carb 45 calorie Sara Lee bread

3 oz turkey

½ T. light mayo

Lettuce, tomato, onion

Make a half turkey sandwich and add lettuce, tomato and onion

Berries 'n' Cream

½ c. low fat cottage cheese

½ c. strawberries

Cinnamon and stevia, to taste

Stir berries into cottage cheese and top with cinnamon and stevia

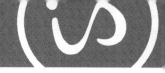

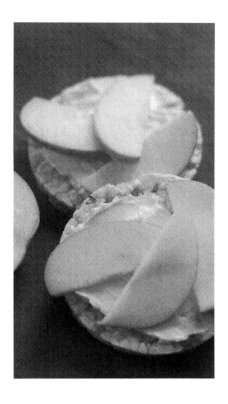

Apple Swiss Rice Cakes

2 wedges light Laughing Cow cheese

½ small granny smith apple, thinly sliced

1 lightly salted rice cake

Spread the cheese over the rice cake and top with apple slices

....

Cheese and Crackers

½ serving whole wheat crackers

1 string cheese

Fruit and Jerky

1 plum

1 oz beef jerky

....

Cheesy Rice Cake Snack

1 cheddar rice cake

½ c. low fat cottage cheese

Top the rice cake with cottage cheese

....

Easy Cheesecake

¾ c. plain fat free Greek yogurt

1 T. sugar free cheesecake pudding powder

½ c. plain cheerios

Sautee the cheerios on a pan over medium heat with spray butter and salt. Stir often. When they're lightly toasted cool in a bowl

Stir stevia and pudding powder into the Greek yogurt.

Top the yogurt with the cheerios and enjoy!

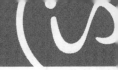

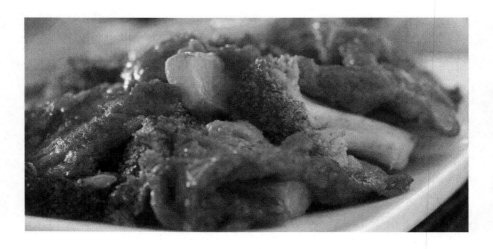

Beef and Broccoli Stir Fry

3 oz lean beef such as Top Sirloin, Flank or London Broil, sliced into thin slices

½ t. minced garlic

¼ t. ginger

½ T. light soy sauce

1 c. broccoli

1 t. coconut oil

1 T. water

6 T. beef broth

½ T. cornstarch

¼ c. bean sprouts, optional

1 T. peanuts, chopped

1. Combine beef, garlic, ginger and soy sauce in a bowl and let stand.

2. Wash broccoli thoroughly and cut into florets.

3. Heat 1 t. oil in a nonstick skillet over high heat, add broccoli and stir fry for 2 minutes. Add water and stir until the water evaporates. Move broccoli to a separate bowl.

4. Heat remaining 2 t. oil, and add beef mixture. Stir fry for 3 minutes. Stir together broth and cornstarch, add to meat and stir fry until sauce is thickened, about 3 more minutes.

5. Add broccoli and bean sprouts, then cook, stirring, until heated through, about 2 more minutes.

6. Top with 1 T. chopped peanuts and enjoy!

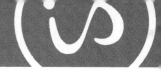

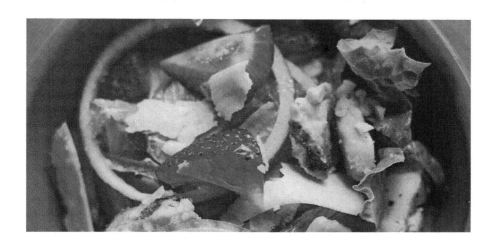

Maple Chicken Salad

Salad:

3 oz chicken, cooked and cut into strips

Romaine Lettuce

Red onion, thinly sliced

5 large strawberries

½ oz swiss cheese, shredded

1 slice turkey bacon, cooked and crumbled

Dressing:

1 t. extra virgin olive oil

1 T. vinegar

1 t. light mayo

½ T. sugar free maple syrup

Stevia to taste, if needed

1. *Combine dressing ingredients and allow to sit for 15-30 minutes in the fridge.*

2. *Meanwhile combine salad ingredients.*

3. *Toss salad in dressing and enjoy!*

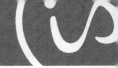

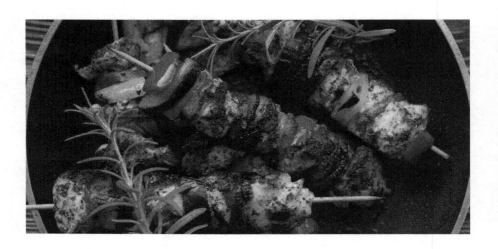

Shish-Ka-Bobs

4 oz chicken, diced

Whole bell pepper, any color, diced

Sweet onion, diced

Cherry tomatoes

Zucchini, diced

⅓ avocado, sliced

Wooden skewers

1. Soak diced, raw chicken in balsamic vinegar for 30 minutes in the fridge.

2. Assemble zucchini, tomatoes, onion, pepper and chicken on wooden skewers.

3. Grill over medium heat until chicken is cooked through.

4. Enjoy shish-ka-bobs with sliced avocado.

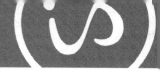

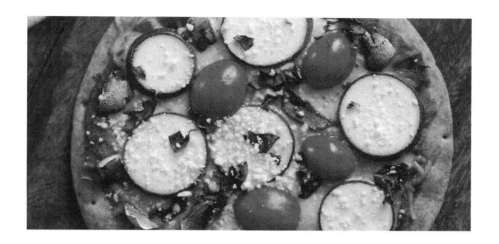

Low Carb Grilled Chicken Pizza

½ zucchini, thinly sliced

2 mushrooms, sliced

1 small corn tortilla (approx 50 cals)

2-3 T. tomato basil pizza sauce

1 oz low fat mozzarella cheese

4 cherry tomatoes

4 oz chicken, cooked and sliced

1 T. fresh basil, chopped

1. *Preheat oven to 180 degrees.*

2. *Grill or roast zucchini and mushrooms until desired tenderness.* Transfer to a plate.*

3. *Place tortilla on a baking tray lined with foil. Spread sauce over tortilla and sprinkle with ½ oz of cheese. Top with grilled veggies, tomatoes and chicken. Top with remaining cheese.*

4. *Bake for 12-15 minutes or until tortilla is crisp and cheese is melted. Sprinkle with basil and serve with a side salad.*

*To grill veggies preheat gas grill over medium heat. Spray the veggies with spray butter or cooking spray and lightly salt them. Cook over low-med heat for approx 5-8 minutes or until desired tenderness is reached. To roast veggies preheat oven to 400 degrees and bake on a baking sheet for approx 20-25 minute or until desired tenderness is reached. Then let oven cool before baking pizza.

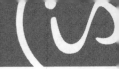

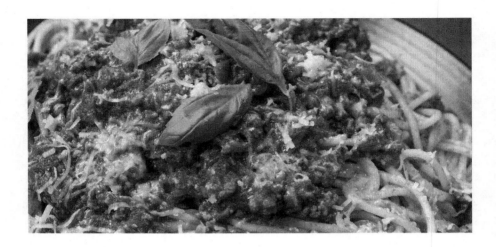

Creamy Bolognese Over Spaghetti Squash

¼ yellow onion, chopped

½ clove garlic

3 oz extra lean ground beef

½ c. pre-made spaghetti sauce

¼ can (14 oz) diced tomatoes, undrained

1 T. light Italian salad dressing

1 T. fat free cream cheese

¼ t. dried basil

¾ c. Spaghetti Squash, cooked and shredded*

1 oz fresh Parmesan cheese

1. Sautee onions in a large skillet on medium heat until they begin to be translucent. Add meat and cook until cooked through, stirring frequently. Drain any excess grease from pan.

2. Stir in spaghetti sauce and tomatoes. Bring to a boil. Reduce heat to medium-low and simmer 15 minutes. Remove from heat and stir in cream cheese, seasonings and Italian salad dressing. Serve hot over cooked spaghetti squash noodles. Top with parmesan cheese.

*To prepare your spaghetti squash in advance start by slicing it half lengthwise. If it's too hard to cut, microwave the whole squash for a few minutes until the skin is soft enough to cut with a large knife. Preheat oven to 375 degrees. Scoop out seeds with a large spoon. Place squash cut side up on a heavy duty baking pan. Roast for 45-50 minutes or until a fork can easily puncture the flesh. Remove squash from the oven and allow to cool until you can handle it, about 3-4 minutes. Scrape the flesh from the squash with a fork until it turns into "noodles" and place in separate bowl to use in your recipe.

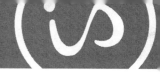

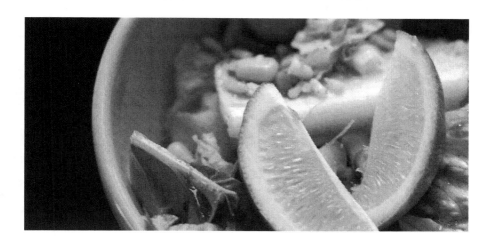

Garlic Lime Chicken Salad

3 T. low sodium soy sauce

1 T. lime juice

2 t. Worcestershire sauce

1 clove garlic

½ t. dry mustard ½ t. pepper

3 oz Chicken breast

1-2 cups romaine lettuce, chopped Green onion, diced

2 T. Corn

5 Cherry tomatoes, halved

2 T. Peas

1 stick celery, diced

1 oz feta cheese

1. *Combine the first six ingredients for your sauce. Reserve 1 T. of the sauce for salad dressing.*

2. *Marinate chicken in the rest of the sauce for 15-30 minutes and grill.*

3. *Meanwhile assemble salad ingredients. Toss salad with veggies, cheese and reserved sauce. Top with chicken.*

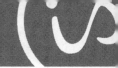

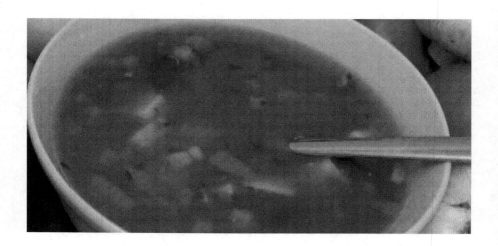

Vegetable Beef Soup

4 oz extra lean ground beef

¼ can (14.5 oz) stewed tomatoes, undrained, cut up

¼ (14 oz) can beef broth

¼ can (8 oz) no salt added tomato sauce

1 c. frozen mixed veggies

¼ avocado

1. *Brown ground beef and drain. In saucepan combine all ingredients and heat to boiling. Reduce heat to medium. Cover and cook 10-15 minutes, stirring occasionally until vegetables are tender. Top with avocado.*

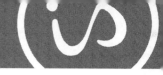

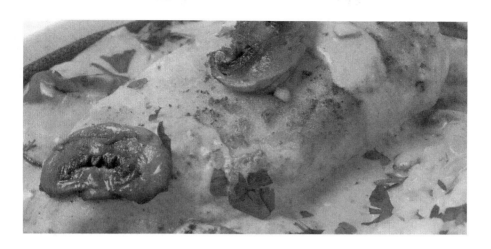

Creamy Crock Pot Chicken

3 oz Chicken breast

¼ can cream of chicken soup

4 sliced mushrooms

½ garlic cloves, pressed

¼ t. Worcestershire sauce

¼ t. lemon juice

1 slice turkey bacon, cooked
    and crumbled

¼ t. vinegar

1 oz cheddar cheese

1. *Combine all ingredients except cheese and chicken breast in a mixing bowl and mix well.*

2. *Put chicken into a crockpot. Cover with soup mixture.*

3. *Cook on low 4-6 hours or until cooked through.*

4. *While still hot top with shredded cheese and allow to melt. Serve with steamed veggies.*

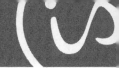

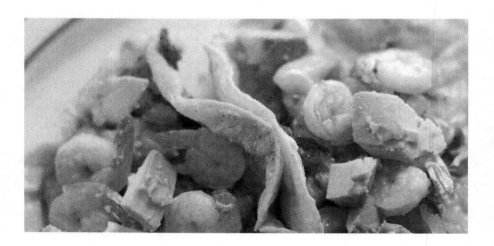

Honey Lime Shrimp Toss

4 oz shrimp

¼ mango

1-2 c. chopped cabbage

Cilantro

Red onion

1 t. honey

1 lime

¼ avocado

1 t. coconut oil

1. *Preheat pan and add 1 t. coconut oil.*

2. *Cook shrimp for 2-3 minutes.*

3. *Drizzle honey and squeeze the juice of half a lime onto the shrimp. Cook for another 3-4 minutes or until cooked through.*

4. *Meanwhile, dice mango and red onion and chop cilantro.*

5. *Toss a salad together with cabbage, mango, onion, cilantro, avocado and shrimp. Drizzle with leftover sauce.*

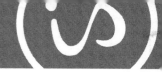

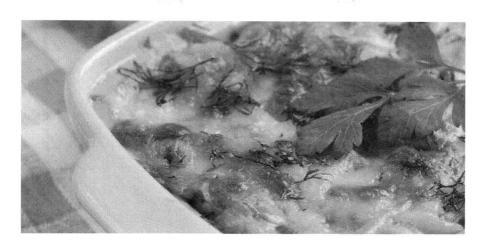

"Breakfast" Casserole

1 turkey sausage

½ oz low fat mozzarella cheese, shredded

½ oz low fat cheddar cheese, shredded

1 T. chopped onion

1 T. chopped bell pepper

½ c. egg beaters

¼ c. milk

Salt and pepper to taste

1 slice turkey bacon

1. *Cook sausage according to package directions. Cool slightly and cut into slices.*

2. *Layer sausage, cheese, onion and bell pepper in a greased single serving baking dish.*

3. *In a separate bowl combine eggs, milk, salt and pepper. Pour over the sausage and cheese mixture.*

4. *Top with crumbled bacon. Cover and refrigerate overnight.*

5. *Bake at 350 degrees for about 25 minutes or until a toothpick inserted in the center comes out clean. Let stand for 5 minutes before eating.*

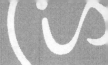

WOMEN 140 lbs - 190 lbs

If you're a woman currently weighing 140-190 lbs, here is everything you need to put IdealPlan into action today! This meal plan is targeted to your gender and body weight range to help you reach your goals faster.

Remember: Make sure to use the recipes and food lists that go with your specific meal plan. The calorie amounts and portions of each macronutrient (carbs, proteins and fats) are slightly different for each weight/gender category.

This program is simple on purpose: we've done all the math for you, giving you the calorie amount and balance of carbs, proteins and fats that are generally ideal for fat loss for your weight range. We've also selected foods that fit great with this template, but if you prefer to use your own comparable substitutions, that's fine too!

Because everybody is different and physical activity levels vary from person to person, you can use the check-in points at the end of Phase 1 and Phase 2 (see FAQ) to adjust the plan according to your results.

Bookmark the next 4 pages for daily reference!

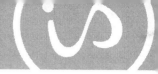

Five-Meal Template

Breakfast Smoothie

1 scoop IdealShake

1 large serving fruit (see fruit list)

1 Protein A Serving

1 c. any milk (see milk list)

Or: choose from the recipes that follow

Mid-Morning Snack

1 IdealBar

Or: 1 Protein A List Option

1 Carb B List Option

Lunch Smoothie

1 scoop IdealShake

1 Carb D serving

1 Fat A serving

1 c. any milk

Or: choose from the recipes that follow

Mid-Afternoon Snack

1 Protein A List Option

1 Carb B List Option

Or: choose from the recipes that follow

Optional: 1 IdealBoost stick pack

Dinner

1 serving any lean meat - (3-4 oz approx size of your palm)

1 Fat B List

1 Carb C List Serving Unlimited vegetables*

Or: choose from the recipes that follow

Approximate daily calories: **1500**

40% carbs | 30% proteins | 30% fats

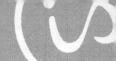

Food Lists

Milk Options
Almond Milk

Soy Milk

Skim Milk

Low fat Milk

Unsweetened Coconut Milk

Coconut Water

Rice Milk

Fruit Servings
1 banana

1 apple

1 orange

1 peach

1 pear

1 mango

1 tangerines 2 apricots

1 kiwis

1 c. berries/cherries/pineapple

1 ½ c. any melon (watermelon, cantaloupe, honeydew, etc)

1 ½ c. grapes

1 c. any fruit juice/veggie juice Or: Any fruit for approx 100 calories

Carb B List (Small Snacks)
1 flavored rice cake

½ c. low sugar cereal (Plain cheerios, Rice Chex, Wheaties, etc)

1 low fat graham cracker

½ serving whole wheat crackers

½ serving pop chips/baked chips

½ serving fruit (see fruit list)

Or: Any low fat carb for approx 50 calories

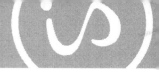
Carb C List (Dinner Options)

½ c. brown/white rice

½ c. couscous

½ c. quinoa

½ c. whole wheat pasta

1 small sweet/red/white potato

1 small whole wheat tortilla

2 corn tortillas

1 slice whole wheat bread

1 serving fruit

Or: Any low fat carb for approx 100 calories

Carb D Options (Shake Add Ins)

½ c. oats

2 T. chia seeds

1 fruit serving (see fruit list)

4 T. PB2 peanut butter powder

2 T. Honey/Agave/Real Maple Syrup

½ c. Plain cheerios (stirred in)

1 flavored yogurt

2 low fat graham crackers

Or: Any low fat carb for approx 150 calories

Protein A Servings (Shake Add Ins/Snack Options)

½ c. low fat cottage cheese

¾ c. fat free plain Greek yogurt

½ scoop whey protein

1 80-100 calorie flavored Greek yogurt (e.g., Dannon Light n Fit Greek)

¾ c. liquid egg whites (can be added to shakes to make it smooth and creamy)

1 egg (hard boiled is easily transportable)

1 oz beef jerky

3 oz turkey slices

1 low fat string cheese 1 serving tuna

Or: Any protein for approx 100 calories

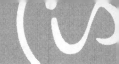

Fat A Serving (Shake Add Ins)

1 T. peanut butter

½ avocado

2 T. flax seed

1 T. coconut oil

3 T. Coconut flakes

½ oz dark chocolate

Or: Any low sugar fat for approx 100 calories

Fat B List (Dinner Options)

1 oz cheese

1 T. any nuts/seeds/nut butter c. feta cheese

1 T. any oil (coconut, extra virgin olive oil, grapeseed oil, etc)

1 T. any salad dressing

½ avocado

Or: Any low sugar fat for approx 100 calories

Freebie Shake Add Ins

2 T. Sugar free fat free pudding powder

1 T. Cocoa Powder

Any Extracts - vanilla, coconut, almond, maple, orange, etc Sugar Free Syrups (e.g., Torani and DaVinci)

¼ t. Crystal Light mix

Any Vegetables*

*Vegetable Cheat Sheet

Fibrous veggies are allowed with any meal in any amount (e.g., asparagus, broccoli, Brussels sprouts, cabbage, cauliflower, celery, okra, cucumber, eggplant, collard greens, tomato, leek, lettuce, any mushroom, green onion, onion, bell pepper, radish, snow peas, spinach, zucchini, fennel, green beans, pickles).

Carrots, peas and squash are not "free" veggies but can be enjoyed occasionally.

Corn and potatoes are counted as grains/carbs in the meal plan.

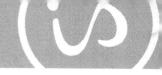

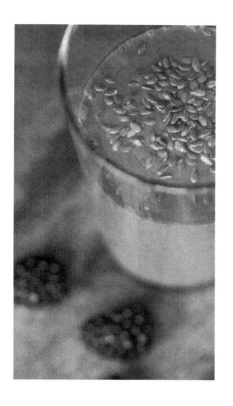

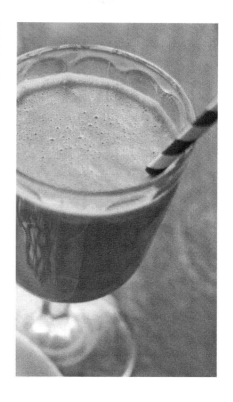

Black Berry Boost

1 scoop Vanilla IdealShake

1 c. unsweetened almond milk

1 c. fresh blackberries

½ c. low fat cottage cheese

Ice Cubes

Chocolate Banana

1 scoop Chocolate IdealShake

1 c. unsweetened almond milk

1 banana

¾ c. plain fat free Greek yogurt

Ice Cubes

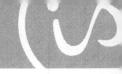

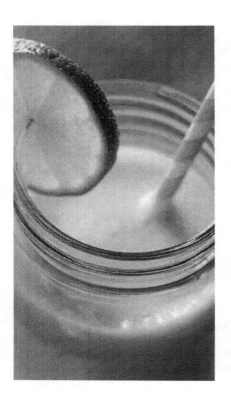

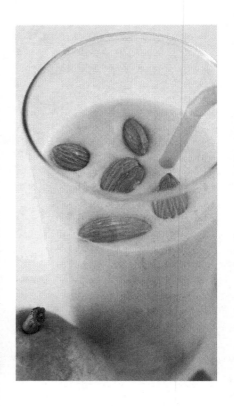

Key Lime Pie

1 scoop Vanilla IdealShake

1 unsweetened almond milk

1 T. lime juice

1 low fat graham cracker*

½ c. low fat cottage cheese

Ice Cubes

*Graham cracker subs for the fruit in
your breakfast shake*

Almond Pear Spice

1 scoop Vanilla IdealShake

1 c. unsweetened almond milk

½ c. low fat cottage cheese

½ banana

½ pear

1 t. cinnamon

1 t. almond extract

Ice Cubes

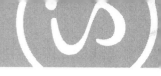

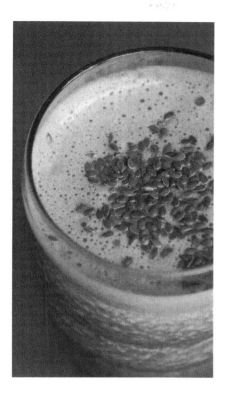

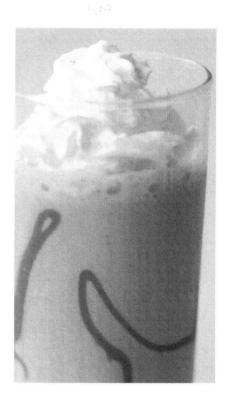

Tropical Greens

1 scoop Vanilla IdealShake

1 c. coconut water

¾ c. plain fat free Greek yogurt

½ c. strawberries

½ c. pineapple

1 c. spinach

Ice Cubes

Salted Caramel Pumpkin Latte

1 scoop Mocha or Vanilla IdealShake [1]

½ cup coffee, cooled

½ c. unswt almond milk

½ c. low fat cottage cheese

2 T. canned pumpkin

½ banana

1-2 T. sugar free Torani Salted
    Caramel Syrup

Pinch of sea salt

Ice Cubes

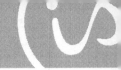

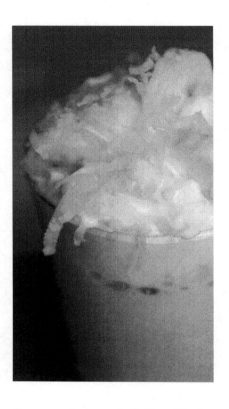

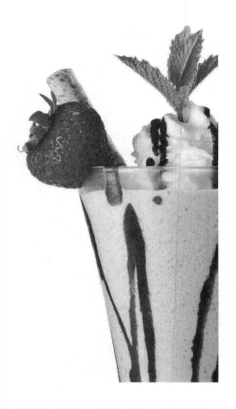

Banana Coconut Coffee Shake

1 scoop Mocha IdealShake

1 c. unswt coconut milk

1 banana

1 container Coconut Dannon Light n Fit Greek Yogurt

1-2 T. sugar free Torani Coconut Syrup

Ice Cubes

Triple Chocolate Berry Shake

1 scoop Chocolate IdealShake

1 c. Hood Carb Countdown Chocolate Milk

¾ c. frozen strawberries

½ c. low fat cottage cheese

2 T. sugar free chocolate pudding powder

Ice Cubes

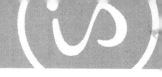

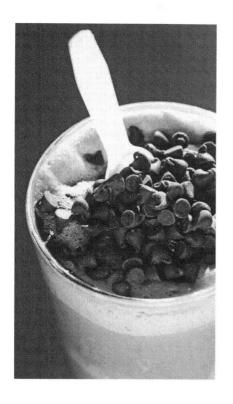

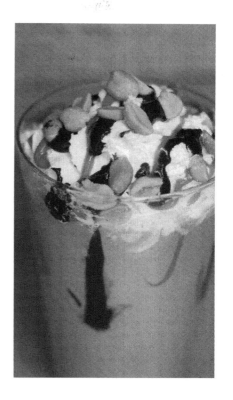

Minty Mocha Shake

1 scoop Mocha IdealShake

½ c. unsweetened almond milk or
   cooled coffee

¾ c. liquid egg whites

½ t. peppermint extract

Ice Cubes

Have one piece of fruit on the side.

Candybar Shake

1 scoop Chocolate IdealShake

1 c. unsweetened almond milk

½ c. low fat cottage cheese

2 T. PB2 peanut butter powder
   (in place of fruit in template)

1 t. cocoa powder

2 t. sugar free caramel syrup

Ice Cubes

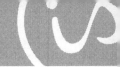

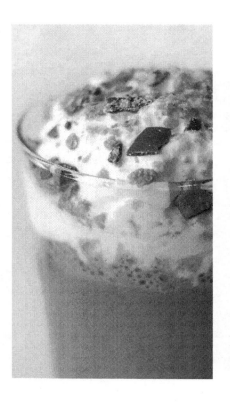

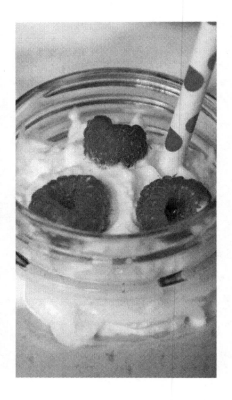

The Butter-Finger

1 scoop Chocolate IdealShake

1 c. Hood Carb Countdown Chocolate milk

1 T. peanut butter

1 T. sugar free fat free butterscotch pudding powder

½ c. oats

½ T. unsweetened cocoa

Sweetener to taste

Ice Cubes

Raspberry Cheesecake

1 scoop Vanilla IdealShake

1 c. unsweetened almond milk

1 c. frozen/fresh raspberries

1 graham cracker square

½ oz dark chocolate*

2 T. cottage cheese

Ice cubes

Dark chocolate can be sprinkled over the top or blended in

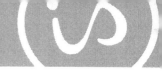

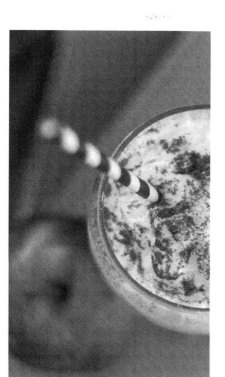

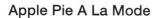

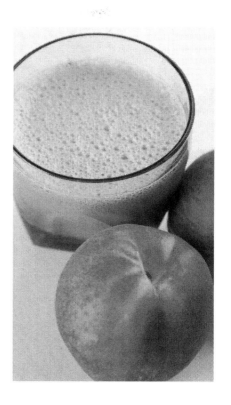

Apple Pie A La Mode

1 scoop Vanilla IdealShake

1 c. unsweetened almond milk

½ c. unsweetened applesauce

2 T. vanilla Greek yogurt

½ t. apple pie spice

¼ c. oats*

1 T. peanut butter

Ice Cubes

Sprinkle the oats over the top of the shake

Peachy Greens

1 scoop Vanilla IdealShake

½ c. water

½ c. orange juice

1 peach, pitted

⅓ avocado

1 c. spinach

Ice cubes

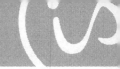

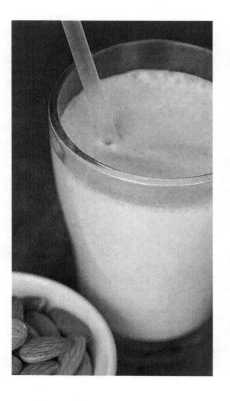

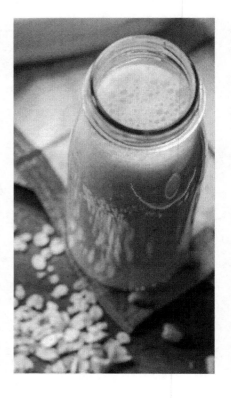

Honey Nut

1 scoop Vanilla IdealShake

1 c. unsweetened almond milk

3 T. PB2 peanut butter powder

1 T. honey

1 T. Almond butter

Ice Cubes

Peanut Butter Cookie

1 scoop Chocolate or Vanilla
  IdealShake

1 c. unswt almond milk

½ c. oats

1 T. peanut butter

Ice Cubes

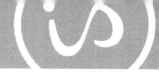

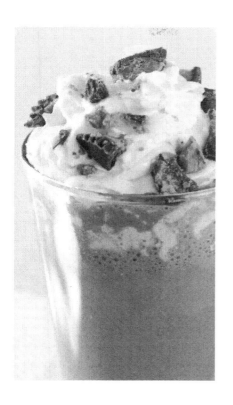

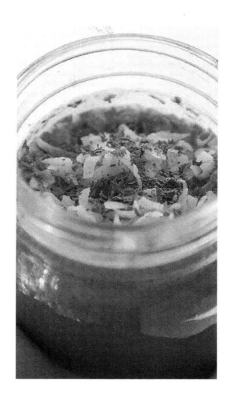

Chocolate Peanut Butter Cup

1 scoop Chocolate IdealShake

1 c. unswt almond milk

4 T. PB2 peanut butter powder

1 T. Peanut butter

Ice Cubes

Almond Delight

1 scoop Chocolate IdealShake

1 c. dark chocolate almond milk

½ c. oats

¼ c. part skim ricotta

1 T. coconut flakes

Ice Cubes

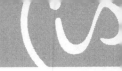

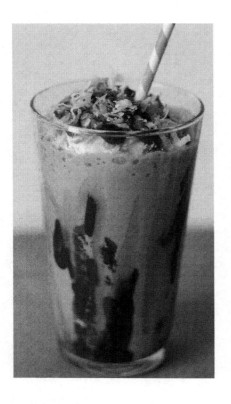

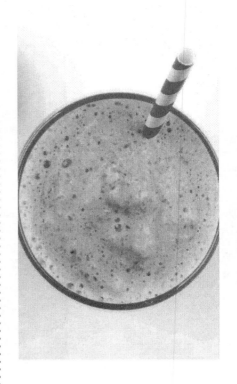

Caramel Coconut Cookie

1 scoop Chocolate IdealShake

1 c. unswt coconut milk

¼ t. coconut extract

2 T. sugar free caramel syrup ice cream topping

2 T. sugar free chocolate syrup ice cream topping

1 T. coconut oil, melted*

Ice Cubes

*Melt the coconut oil and then drizzle slowly into shake while blender is mixing to prevent clumping.

Berries n Cream

1 scoop Strawberry IdealShake

1 c. unswt almond milk

½ c. frozen raspberries

½ c. frozen strawberries

2 T. sugar free french vanilla creamer

1 T. fat free sugar free vanilla pudding mix

1 T. flax seeds

Ice Cubes

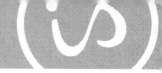

Optional:

1 IdealBoost Stick Pack drink on the side with your snack!

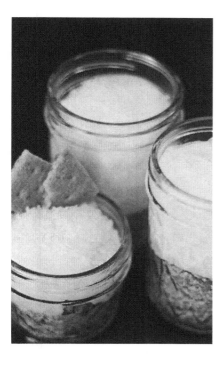

Coconut Cream Pie

1 container Coconut Dannon Light n Fit Greek yogurt

1 low fat graham cracker, crumbled

* Stir graham cracker crumbs into yogurt

Tuna "Sandwich"

3 oz tuna

½ T. light mayo

1 lightly salted rice cake

*Mix tuna and mayo and spread over the rice cake

Easy Cheesecake

¾ c. plain fat free Greek yogurt

1 T. sugar free cheesecake pudding powder

½ c. plain cheerios

*Sautee the cheerios on a pan over medium heat with spray butter and salt. Stir often. When they're lightly toasted cool in a bowl.

*Stir stevia and pudding powder into the Greek yogurt.

*Top the yogurt with the cheerios and enjoy!

Berries 'n' Cream

½ c. low fat cottage cheese

½ c. strawberries Cinnamon and stevia, to taste

*Stir berries into cottage cheese and top with cinnamon and stevia

Fruit and Eggs

¾ c. grapes

1 hardboiled egg

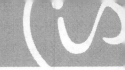

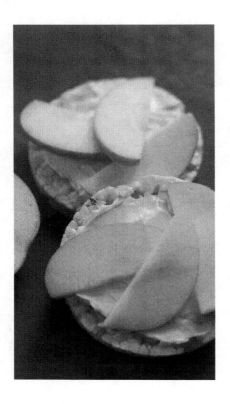

Apple Swiss Rice Cakes

2 wedges light Laughing Cow cheese

½ small granny smith apple, thinly sliced

1 lightly salted rice cake

Spread the cheese over the rice cake and top with apple slices

Turkey Sandwich

1 slice low carb 45 calorie Sara Lee bread 3 oz turkey

½ T. light mayo Lettuce, tomato, onion

*Make a half turkey sandwich and add lettuce tomato and onion

Cheese and Crackers

½ serving whole wheat crackers

1 string cheese

Cheesy Rice Cake Snack

1 cheddar rice cake

½ c. low fat cottage cheese

*Top the rice cake with cottage cheese

Fruit and Jerky

1 plum

1 oz beef jerky

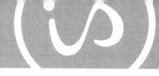

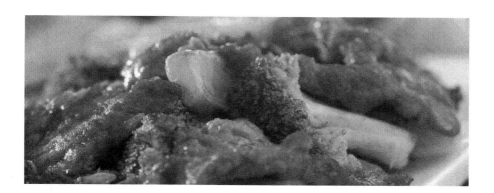

Beef and Broccoli Stir Fry

3 oz lean beef such as Top Sirloin, Flank or London Broil, sliced into thin slices

½ t. minced garlic

¼ t. ginger

½ T. light soy sauce

1 c. broccoli

½ T. coconut oil

2 T. water

6 T. beef broth

½ T. cornstarch

¼ c. bean sprouts, optional

1 T. peanuts, chopped

½ c. brown rice, cooked

1. Combine beef, garlic, ginger and soy sauce in a bowl and let stand.

2. Wash broccoli thoroughly and cut into florets.

3. Heat 1 t. oil in a nonstick skillet over high heat, add broccoli and stir fry for 2 minutes. Add water and stir until the water evaporates. Move broccoli to a separate bowl.

4. Heat remaining 2 t. oil, and add beef mixture. Stir fry for 3 minutes. Stir together broth and cornstarch, add to meat and stir fry until sauce is thickened, about 3 more minutes.

5. Add broccoli and bean sprouts, then cook, stirring, until heated through, about 2 more minutes.

6. Top with 1 T. chopped peanuts, spread over ½ c. brown rice and enjoy!

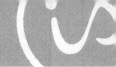

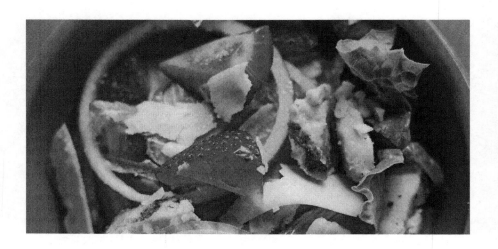

Maple Chicken Salad

Salad:

1 oz chicken, cooked and cut into strips

Romaine Lettuce

Red onion, thinly sliced

5 large strawberries

½ oz swiss cheese, shredded

1 slice turkey bacon, cooked and crumbled

½ c. quinoa, cooked

Dressing:

1 t. extra virgin olive oil

1 T. vinegar

1 t. light mayo

½ T. sugar free maple syrup Stevia to taste, if needed

1. Combine dressing ingredients and allow to sit for 15-30 minutes in the fridge.

2. Meanwhile combine salad ingredients.

3. Toss salad in dressing and enjoy!

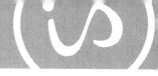

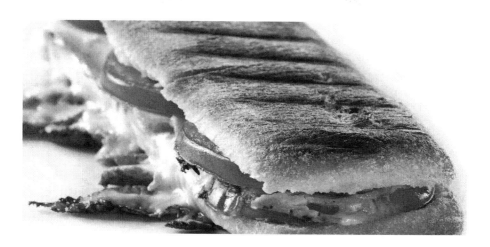

Balsamic Chicken Panini

4 oz chicken

½ c. Balsamic Vinegar

Whole bell pepper, thinly sliced

Sweet onion, thinly sliced

¼ avocado, sliced

½ oz provolone cheese, sliced

Whole Wheat Sandwich Thin

1. *Slice chicken breast in half so that it's cut thinly. Sautee in ¼ c. vinegar until cooked through.*

2. *Place chicken in a separate bowl. Sautee peppers and onion in ¼ c. vinegar until soft and cooked through.*

3. *Spray both sides of the sandwich thin with spray butter and assemble sandwich with chicken, veggies, avocado and cheese.*

4. *Grill the sandwich on an indoor grill (ie George Foreman) or on the stove in a pan over medium heat.*

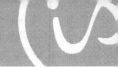

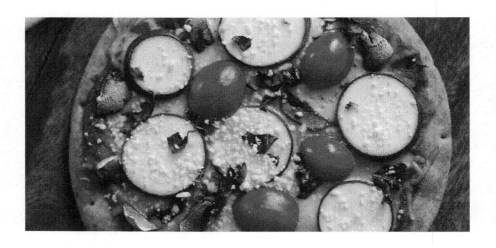

Low Carb Grilled Chicken Pizza

½ zucchini, thinly sliced

2 mushrooms, sliced

1 pita or whole wheat tortilla (approx 100 calories)

2-3 T. tomato basil pizza sauce

1 ½ oz low fat mozzarella cheese

4 cherry tomatoes

4 oz chicken, cooked and sliced

1 T. fresh basil, chopped

1. *Preheat oven to 180 degrees.*

2. *Grill or roast zucchini and mushrooms until desired tenderness.* Transfer to a plate.*

3. *Place tortilla on a baking tray lined with foil. Spread sauce over tortilla and sprinkle with ½ oz of cheese. Top with grilled veggies, tomatoes and chicken. Top with remaining cheese.*

4. *Bake for 12-15 minutes or until tortilla is crisp and cheese is melted. Sprinkle with basil and serve with a side salad.*

*To grill veggies preheat gas grill over medium heat. Spray the veggies with spray butter or cooking spray and lightly salt them. Cook over low-med heat for approx 5-8 minutes or until desired tenderness is reached. To roast veggies preheat oven to 400 degrees and bake on a baking sheet for approx 20-25 minute or until desired tenderness is reached. Then let oven cool before baking pizza.

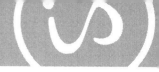

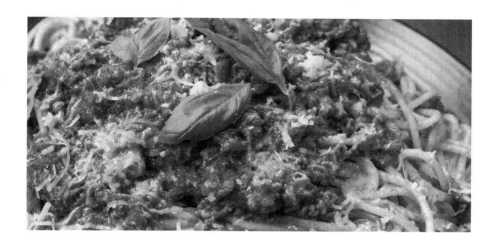

Creamy Bolognese over Spaghetti

¼ yellow onion, chopped

½ clove garlic

4 oz extra lean ground beef

½ c. premade spaghetti sauce

¼ can (14 oz) diced tomatoes, undrained

1 T. Light Italian Salad Dressing

1 T. fat free cream cheese

¼ t. dried basil

1 oz whole wheat spaghetti noodles, dry

1 oz fresh Parmesan cheese

1. Sautee onions in a large skillet on medium heat until they begin to be translucent. Add meat and cook until cooked through, stirring frequently. Drain any excess grease from pan.

2. Meanwhile cook spaghetti noodles.

3. Stir in spaghetti sauce and tomatoes. Bring to a boil. Reduce heat to medium-low and simmer 15 minutes. Remove from heat and stir in cream cheese, seasonings and Italian salad dressing. Serve hot over cooked spaghetti noodles. Top with parmesan cheese.

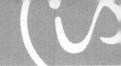

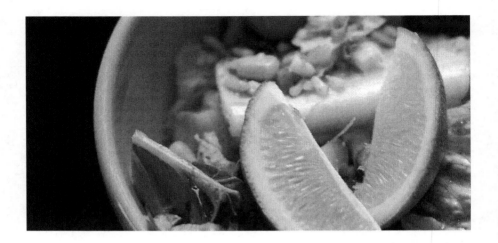

Garlic Lime Chicken Salad

3 T. low sodium soy sauce

1 T. lime juice

2 t. Worcestershire sauce

1 clove garlic

½ t. dry mustard ½ t. pepper

4 oz Chicken breast

1-2 cups romaine lettuce, chopped
   Green onion, diced

¼ c. Corn

5 Cherry tomatoes, halved

½ c. Peas

1 stick celery, diced

1 oz feta cheese

⅓ c. brown rice

1. *Combine the first six ingredients for your sauce. Reserve 1 T. of the sauce for salad dressing.*

2. *Marinate chicken in the rest of the sauce for 15-30 minutes and grill.*

3. *Meanwhile assemble salad ingredients. Toss salad with rice, veggies, cheese and reserved sauce. Top with chicken.*

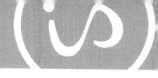

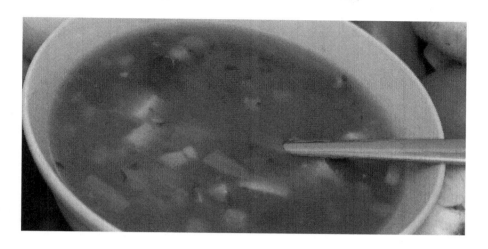

Vegetable, Beef and Barley Stew

4 oz extra lean ground beef

¼ can (14.5 oz) stewed tomatoes, undrained, cut up

¼ (14 oz) can beef broth

¼ can (8 oz) no salt added tomato sauce

1 c. frozen mixed veggies

3 T. quick cooking barley

¼ avocado

1. *Brown ground beef and drain. In saucepan combine all ingredients and heat to boiling. Reduce heat to medium. Cover and cook 10-15 minutes, stirring occasionally until vegetables and barley are tender. Top with avocado.*

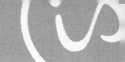

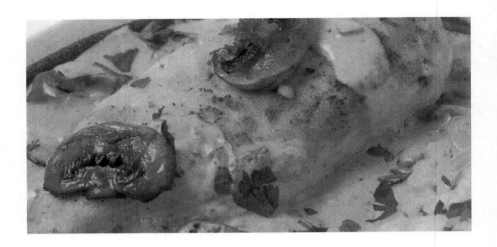

Creamy Crock Pot Chicken

3 oz Chicken breast

½ can cream of chicken soup

4 Sliced mushrooms

½ garlic cloves, pressed

¼ t. Worcestershire sauce

¼ t. lemon juice

1 slice turkey bacon, cooked and crumbled

¼ t. vinegar

1 oz cheddar cheese

½ c. white rice, prepared

1. Combine all ingredients except cheese, rice and chicken breast in a mixing bowl and mix well.

2. Put chicken into a crockpot. Cover with soup mixture.

3. Cook on low 4-6 hours or until cooked through.

4. While still hot top with shredded cheese and allow to melt. Serve with ½ c. white rice and steamed veggies.

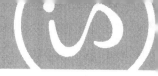

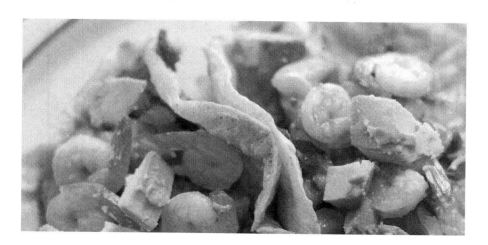

Honey Lime Shrimp Tacos

1 Corn Tortilla

4 oz Shrimp

½ Mango

1-2 c. chopped cabbage

Cilantro

Red Onion

1 t. Honey

1 lime

¼ Avocado

1 t. coconut oil

1. Warm your pan over medium heat and toast corn tortilla until it's slightly crispy.

2. Add 1 t. coconut oil to the pan and cook shrimp for 2-3 minutes.

3. Drizzle honey and squeeze the juice of half a lime onto the shrimp. Cook for another 3-4 minutes or until cooked through.

4. Meanwhile, dice mango and red onion and chop cilantro.

5. Assemble tacos drizzling the sauce over the shrimp. Top with cabbage, mango, onion and avocado.

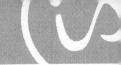

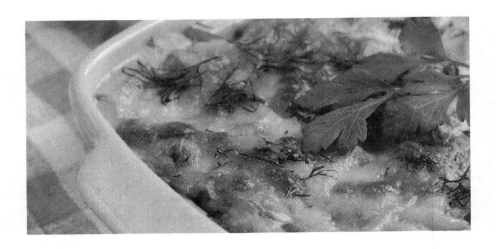

English Muffin Casserole

1 turkey sausage

1 whole wheat English muffin

½ oz low fat mozzarella cheese, shredded

½ oz low fat cheddar cheese, shredded

1 T chopped onion

1 T chopped bell pepper

½ c. egg beaters

¼ c. milk

Salt and pepper to taste

1 slice turkey bacon

1. *Cook sausage according to package directions. Cool slightly and cut into slices.*

2. *Cut English muffin into 1 inch cubes and put in greased single serving baking dish.*

3. *Layer with sausage, cheese, onion and bell pepper.*

4. *In a separate bowl combine eggs, milk, salt and pepper. Pour over the the sausage and cheese mixture.*

5. *Top with crumbled bacon. Cover and refrigerate overnight.*

6. *Remove from the fridge 30 minutes prior to baking. Uncover and bake at 350 degrees for about 30 minutes or until a toothpick inserted in the center comes out clean. Let stand for 5 minutes before eating.*

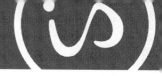

WOMEN OVER 190 lbs

If you're a woman currently weighing over 190 lbs, here is everything you need to put IdealPlan into action today! This meal plan is targeted to your gender and body weight range to help you reach your goals faster.

Remember: Make sure to use the recipes and food lists that go with your specific meal plan. The calorie amounts and portions of each macronutrient (carbs, proteins and fats) are slightly different for each weight/gender category.

This program is simple on purpose: we've done all the math for you, giving you the calorie amount and balance of carbs, proteins and fats that are generally ideal for fat loss for your weight range. We've also selected foods that fit great with this template, but if you prefer to use your own comparable substitutions, that's fine too!

Because everybody is different and physical activity levels vary from person to person, you can use the check-in points at the end of Phase 1 and Phase 2 (see FAQ) to adjust the plan according to your results.

Bookmark the first 4 pages for daily reference!

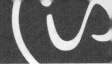

Five-Meal Template

Breakfast Smoothie

1 scoop IdealShake

1 serving fruit (see fruit list)

1 Protein B Serving

1 c. any milk (see milk list)

Or: choose from the recipes that follow

Mid-Morning Snack

1 IdealBar

10 almonds OR 1 string cheese

Or: 1 Protein B List Option

1 Carb B List Option

10 almonds OR 1 string cheese

Lunch Smoothie

1 scoop IdealShake

1 Carb D List Serving

1 Fat C List serving

1 c. any milk

Or: choose from the recipes that follow

Mid-Afternoon Snack

1 Protein B List Serving

1 Carb B List Serving

Or: choose from the recipes that follow

Optional: 1 IdealBoost stick pack

Dinner

1 serving any lean meat - 3-4 oz (approx size of your palm)

1 Fat B List Serving

1 Carb C List Serving

Unlimited vegetables*

Or: choose from the recipes that follow

Approximate daily calories: **1800**

40% carbs | 30% proteins | 30% fats

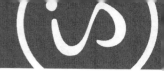

Food Lists

Milk Options

Almond Milk

Soy Milk

Skim Milk

Low fat Milk

Unsweetened Coconut Milk Coconut Water Rice Milk

Fruit Servings

1 banana

1 apple

1 orange

1 peach

1 pear

1 mango

2 tangerines

2 apricots

2 kiwis

1 c. berries/cherries/pineapple

1 ½ c. any melon (watermelon, cantaloupe, honeydew, etc)

1 ½ c. grapes

1 c. any fruit juice/veggie juice Or: Any fruit for approx 100 calories

Carb B List (Small Snacks)

1 flavored rice cake

½ c. low sugar cereal (Plain cheerios, Rice Chex, Wheaties, etc)

1 low fat graham cracker

½ serving whole wheat crackers

½ serving pop chips/baked chips

½ serving fruit (see fruit list)

Or: Any low fat carb for approx 50 calories

OVER 190 lbs

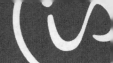

Carb C List (Dinner Options)

½ c. brown/white rice

½ c. couscous

½ c. quinoa

½ c. whole wheat pasta

1 small sweet/red/white potato

1 small whole wheat tortilla

2 corn tortillas

1 slice whole wheat bread

1 serving fruit

Or: Any low fat carb for approx 100 calories

Carb D List (Shake Add-In's)

½ c. oats

2 T. chia seeds

1 fruit serving (see fruit list)

4 T. PB2 peanut butter powder

2 T. Honey/Agave/Real Maple Syrup

½ c. Plain Cheerios stirred in (or other low sugar cereal)

1 flavored yogurt

2 low fat graham crackers

Or: Any low fat carb for approx 150 calories

Protein B Servings (Shake Add-Ins/Snack Options)

¾ c. low fat cottage cheese

1 c. plain fat free Greek yogurt

1 scoop whey protein

150 calorie flavored Greek yogurt (e.g., Chobani)

1 c. liquid egg whites (can be added to shakes to make them smooth and creamy)

2 eggs (hard boiled are easily transportable)

2 oz beef jerky

5 oz Turkey slices

2 low fat string cheese

1 ½ servings tuna

Or: Any protein for approx 150 calories

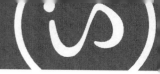

Fat B List (Dinner Options)

1 oz cheese

1 T. any nuts/seeds/nut butter

¼ c. feta cheese

1 T. any oil (coconut, extra virgin olive oil, grapeseed oil, etc)

1 T. any salad dressing % avocado

Or: Any low sugar fat for approx 100 calories

Fat C List (Shake Add-Ins):

2 T. peanut butter ¾ avocado

4 T. flax seed 1 / T. coconut oil 6 T. coconut flakes

1 ½ oz dark chocolate

Or: Any low sugar fat for approx 200 calories

Freebie Shake Add-In's

2 T. Sugar free fat free pudding powder

1 T. Cocoa Powder

Any Extracts - vanilla, coconut, almond, maple, orange, etc Sugar Free Syrups (e.g., Torani and DaVinci)

Sugar Free Syrups (e.g., Torani and DaVinci)

¼ t. Crystal Light mix

Any Vegetables*

---

*Vegetable Cheat Sheet

Fibrous veggies are allowed with any meal in any amount (e.g., asparagus, broccoli, Brussels sprouts, cabbage, cauliflower, celery, okra, cucumber, eggplant, collard greens, tomato, leek, lettuce, any mushroom, green onion, onion, bell pepper, radish, snow peas, spinach, zucchini, fennel, green beans, pickles).

Carrots, peas and squash are not "free" veggies but can be enjoyed occasionally.

Corn and potatoes are counted as grains/carbs in the meal plan.

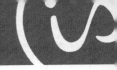

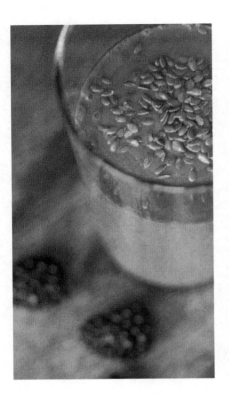

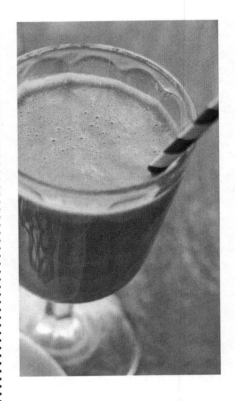

Black Berry Boost

1 scoop Vanilla IdealShake

1 c. unsweetened almond milk

1 c. fresh blackberries

½ c. low fat cottage cheese

⅓ c. liquid egg whites

Ice Cubes

Chocolate Banana

1 scoop Chocolate IdealShake

1 c. unsweetened almond milk

1 banana

1 c. plain fat free Greek yogurt

Ice Cubes

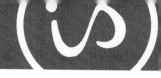

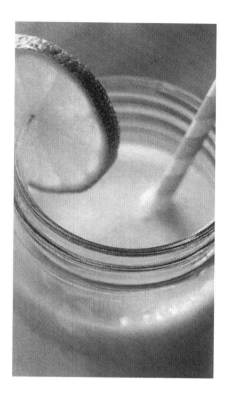

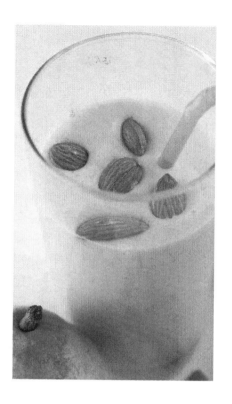

Key Lime Pie

1 scoop Vanilla IdealShake

1 c. unsweetened almond milk

1 T. lime juice

1 low fat graham cracker*

¾ c. low fat cottage cheese

Ice Cubes

Graham cracker subs for the fruit in your breakfast shake

Almond Pear Spice

1 scoop Vanilla IdealShake

¾ c. unsweetened almond milk

⅓ c. liquid egg whites

½ c. low fat cottage cheese

½ banana

½ pear

1 t. cinnamon

1 t. almond extract

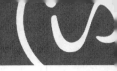

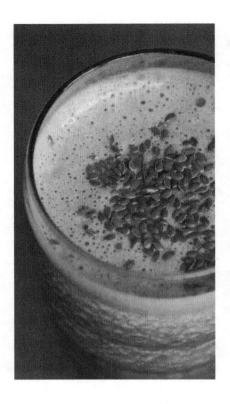

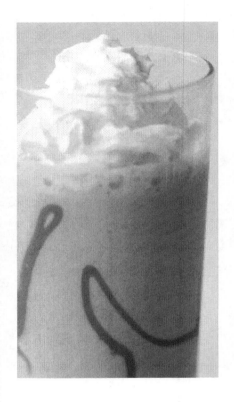

Tropical Greens

1 scoop Vanilla IdealShake

1 c. coconut water

1 c. plain fat free Greek yogurt

½ c. strawberries

½ c. pineapple

1 c. spinach

Ice Cubes

Salted Caramel Pumpkin Latte

1 scoop Mocha or Vanilla IdealShake

½ cup coffee, cooled

½ c. unswt almond milk

¾ c. low fat cottage cheese

2 T. canned pumpkin

½ banana

1-2 T. sugar free Torani Salted Caramel Syrup

Pinch of sea salt

Ice Cubes

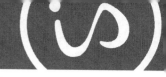

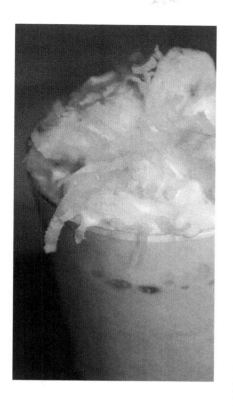

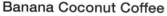

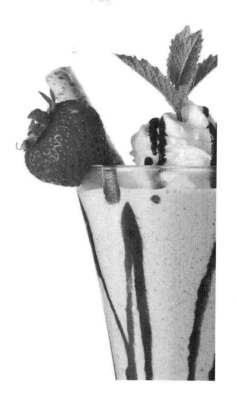

Banana Coconut Coffee

1 scoop Mocha IdealShake

½ c. unswt coconut milk

½ c. liquid egg whites

1 banana

1 container Coconut Dannon Light n
   Fit Greek Yogurt

1-2 T. sugar free Torani Coconut Syrup

Ice Cubes

Triple Chocolate Berry

1 scoop Chocolate IdealShake

1 c. Hood Carb Countdown
   Chocolate Milk

¾ c. frozen strawberries

¾ c. low fat cottage cheese

2 T. sugar free chocolate pudding
   powder

Ice Cubes

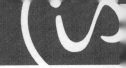

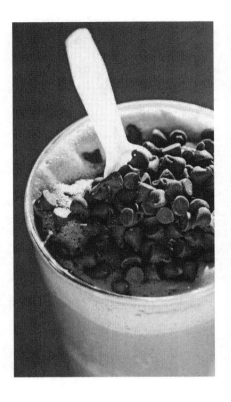

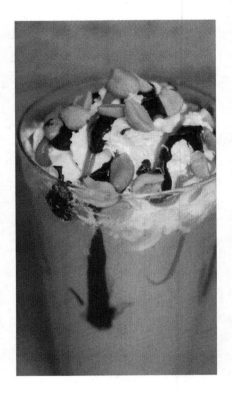

Minty Mocha

1 scoop Mocha IdealShake

¼ c. unsweetened almond milk or
    cooled coffee

1 c. liquid egg whites

½ t. peppermint extract

Ice Cubes

Have one piece of fruit on the side.

Candybar

1 scoop Chocolate IdealShake

1 c. unsweetened almond milk

¾ c. low fat cottage cheese

2 T. PB2 peanut butter powder
    (in place of fruit in template)

1 t. cocoa powder

2 t. sugar free caramel syrup

Ice Cubes

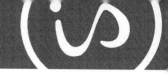

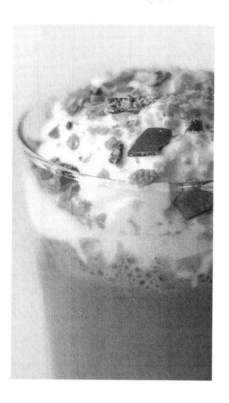

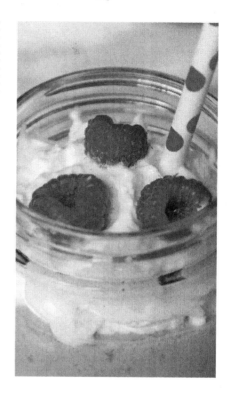

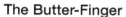

The Butter-Finger

1 scoop Chocolate IdealShake

1 c. Hood Carb Countdown Chocolate Milk

2 T. peanut butter

1 T. sugar free fat free butterscotch pudding powder

½ c. oats

½ T. unsweetened cocoa Sweetener to taste

Ice Cubes

Raspberry Cheesecake

1 scoop Vanilla IdealShake

1 c. unsweetened almond milk

1 c. frozen/fresh raspberries

1 graham cracker sheet

1 oz dark chocolate*

2 T. cottage cheese

Ice cubes

Dark chocolate can be sprinkled over the top or blended in

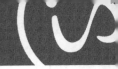

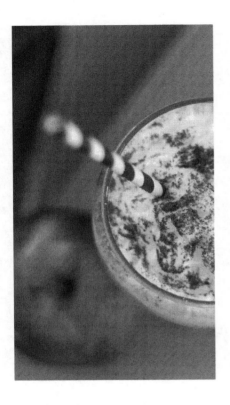

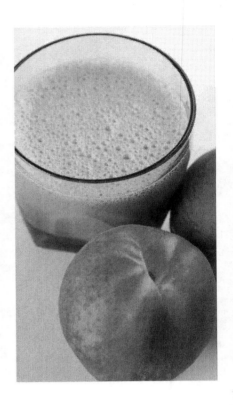

Apple Pie A La Mode

1 scoop Vanilla IdealShake

1 c. unsweetened almond milk

½ c. unsweetened applesauce

¼ c. vanilla Greek yogurt

½ t. apple pie spice

¼ oats*

2 T. peanut butter

Ice Cubes

Blend most of the oats into the shake but save 1-2 T to sprinkle the oats over the top of the shake

Peachy Greens

1 scoop Vanilla IdealShake

¾ c. orange juice

1 peach, pitted

¾ avocado

1 c. spinach

Ice cubes

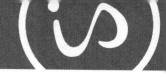

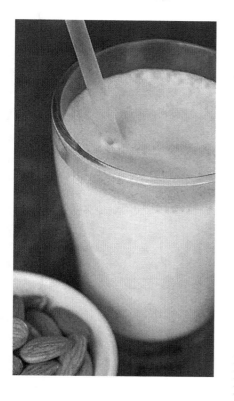

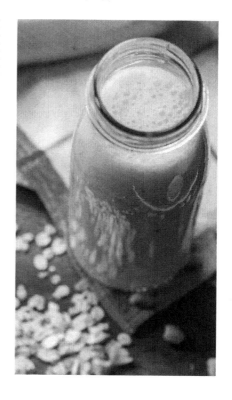

Honey Nut

1 scoop Vanilla IdealShake

1 c. unsweetened almond milk

3 T. PB2 peanut butter powder

1 T. honey

2 T. Almond butter

Ice Cubes

Peanut Butter Cookie

1 scoop Chocolate or Vanilla
IdealShake

1 c. unswt almond milk

½ c. oats

2 T. peanut butter

Ice Cubes

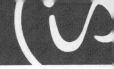

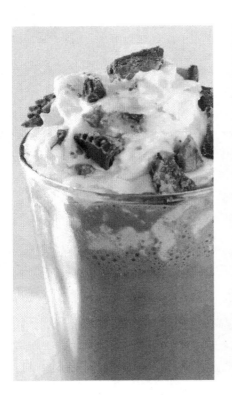

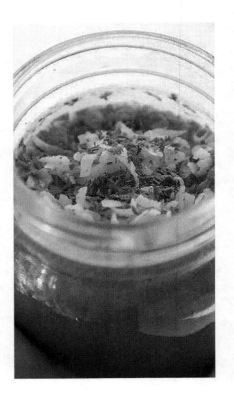

Chocolate Peanut Butter Cup

1 scoop Chocolate IdealShake

1 c. unswt almond milk

3 T. PB2 peanut butter powder

¼ c. oats

2 T. Peanut butter

Ice Cubes

Almond Delight

1 c. dark chocolate almond milk

¼ c. oats

1 T. chia seeds

¼ c. part skim ricotta

1 T. coconut flakes, sprinkled over
the top

12g slivered almonds, sprinkled
over the top

Ice Cubes

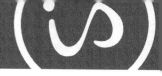

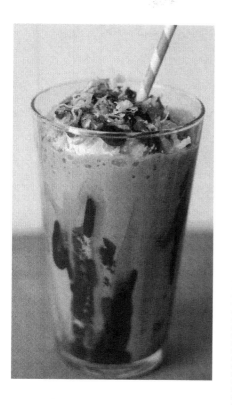

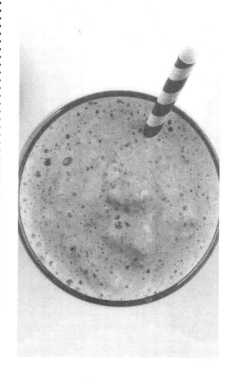

Caramel Coconut Cookie

1 scoop Chocolate IdealShake

1 c. unswt coconut milk

¼ t. coconut extract

2 T. sugar free caramel syrup ice cream

1 T. sugar free chocolate syrup ice cream

2 T. oats

1 T. coconut oil, melted*

1 T. coconut flakes

Ice Cubes

*Melt the coconut oil and then drizzle slowly into shake while blender is mixing to prevent clumping.

Berries n Cream

1 scoop Strawberry IdealShake

1 c. unswt almond milk

½ c. frozen raspberries

½ c. frozen strawberries

2 T. sugar free french vanilla creamer

1 T. fat free sugar free vanilla pudding mix

¼ c. oats

2 T. flax seeds

⅓ avocado

Ice Cubes

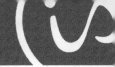

Optional:
1 IdealBoost Stick Pack drink on the side with your snack!

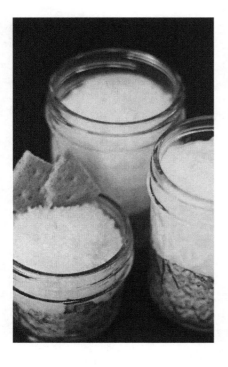

Coconut Cream Pie

1 container Coconut Chobani Greek
  yogurt
1 low fat graham cracker, crumbled

Stir graham cracker crumbs into yogurt.

Berries 'n' Cream

¾ c. low fat cottage cheese

½ c. strawberries

Cinnamon and stevia, to taste

Stir berries into cottage cheese and top with cinnamon and stevia.

Tuna "Sandwich"

3 oz tuna

1 hard boiled egg

½ T. light mayo

1 lightly salted rice cake

Mix tuna and mayo and spread over the rice cake. Have egg on the side or mix into the tuna salad.

Fruit and Eggs

¾ c. grapes

2 hardboiled eggs

Turkey Sandwich

1 slice low carb 45 calorie Sara Lee
  bread

4 oz turkey

½ T. light mayo

Lettuce, tomato, onion

Make a half turkey sandwich and add lettuce tomato and onion.

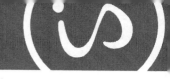

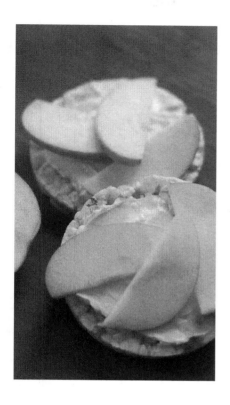

Apple Swiss Rice Cakes

2 wedges light *Laughing Cow* cheese

⅓ c. low fat cottage cheese

¼ small granny smith apple,
thinly sliced

1 lightly salted rice cake

*Spread the cheese over the rice cake
and top with apple slices*

Fruit and Jerky

1 plum

2 oz beef jerky

Cheese and Crackers

½ serving whole wheat crackers

2 string cheese sticks

Cheesy Rice Cake Snack

1 cheddar rice cake

¾ c. low fat cottage cheese

Top the rice cake with cottage cheese.

Easy Cheesecake

½ c. plain fat free Greek yogurt

½ c. low fat cottage cheese

2 T. sugar free cheesecake pudding
powder

½ c. plain cheerios

*Sautee the cheerios on a pan over
medium heat with spray butter and
salt. Stir often. When they're lightly
toasted cool in a bowl.*

*Stir stevia and pudding powder into
the Greek yogurt.*

*Top the yogurt with the cheerios and
enjoy!*

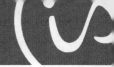

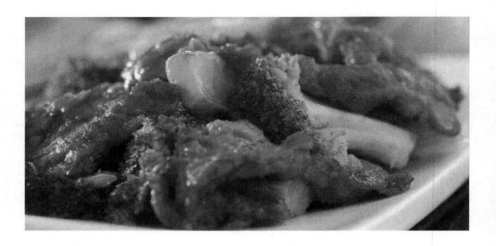

Beef and Broccoli Stir Fry

3 oz lean beef such as Top Sirloin,
   Flank or London Broil,
   sliced into thin slices

½ t. minced garlic

¼ t. ginger

½ T. light soy sauce

1 c. broccoli

½ T. coconut oil

2 T. water

6 T. beef broth

½ T. cornstarch

¼ c. bean sprouts, optional

1 T. peanuts, chopped

½ c. brown rice, cooked

1. Combine beef, garlic, ginger and soy sauce in a bowl and let stand.

2. Wash broccoli thoroughly and cut into florets.

3. Heat 1 t. oil in a nonstick skillet over high heat, add broccoli and stir fry for 2 minutes. Add water and stir until the water evaporates. Move broccoli to a separate bowl.

4. Heat remaining 2 t. oil, and add beef mixture. Stir fry for 3 minutes. Stir together broth and cornstarch, add to meat and stir fry until sauce is thickened, about 3 more minutes.

5. Add broccoli and bean sprouts, then cook, stirring, until heated through, about 2 more minutes.

6. Top with 1 T. chopped peanuts, spread over ½ c. brown rice and enjoy!

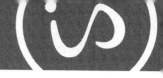

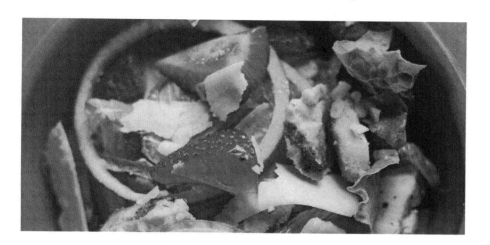

Maple Chicken Salad

Salad:

4 oz chicken, cooked and cut into strips

Romaine Lettuce

Red onion, thinly sliced

5 large strawberries

½ oz swiss cheese, shredded

1 slice turkey bacon, cooked and crumbled

½ c. quinoa, cooked

Dressing:

1 t. extra virgin olive oil

1 T. vinegar

1 t. light mayo

½ T. sugar free maple syrup

Stevia to taste, if needed

1. *Combine dressing ingredients and allow to sit for 15-30 minutes in the fridge.*

2. *Meanwhile combine salad ingredients.*

3. *Toss salad in dressing and enjoy!*

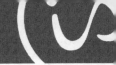

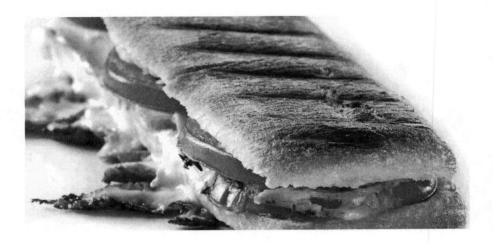

Balsamic Chicken Panini

4 oz chicken

½ c. Balsamic Vinegar

Whole bell pepper, thinly sliced

Sweet onion, thinly sliced

¼ avocado, sliced

½ oz provolone cheese, sliced

Whole Wheat Sandwich Thin

1. Slice chicken breast in half so that it's cut thinly. Sautee in ¼ c. vinegar until cooked through.

2. Place chicken in a separate bowl. Sautee peppers and onion in ¼ c. vinegar until soft and cooked through.

3. Spray both sides of the sandwich thin with spray butter and assemble sandwich with chicken, veggies, avocado and cheese.

4. Grill the sandwich on an indoor grill (ie George Foreman) or on the stove in a pan over medium heat.

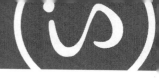

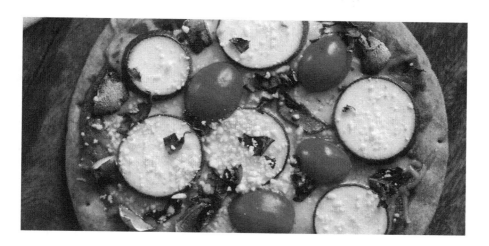

Low Carb Grilled Chicken Pizza

½ zucchini, thinly sliced

2 mushrooms, sliced

1 pita or whole wheat tortilla (approx 100 calories)

2-3 T. tomato basil pizza sauce

1 ½ oz low fat mozzarella cheese

4 cherry tomatoes

4 oz chicken, cooked and sliced

1 T. fresh basil, chopped

1. Preheat oven to 180 degrees.

2. Grill or roast zucchini and mushrooms until desired tenderness.* Transfer to a plate.

3. Place tortilla on a baking tray lined with foil. Spread sauce over tortilla and sprinkle with 1 and ½ oz of cheese. Top with grilled veggies, tomatoes and chicken. Top with remaining cheese.

4. Bake for 12-15 minutes or until tortilla is crisp and cheese is melted. Sprinkle with basil and serve with a side salad.

*To grill veggies preheat gas grill over medium heat. Spray the veggies with spray butter or cooking spray and lightly salt them. Cook over low-med heat for approx 5-8 minutes or until desired tenderness is reached. To roast veggies preheat oven to 400 degrees and bake on a baking sheet for approx 20-25 minute or until desired tenderness is reached. Then let oven cool before baking pizza.

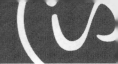

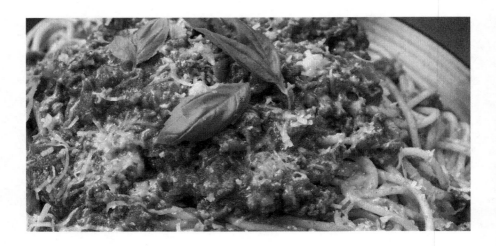

Creamy Bolognese over Spaghetti

¼ yellow onion, chopped

½ clove garlic

4 oz extra lean ground beef

½ c. premade spaghetti sauce

¼ c. (14 oz) diced tomatoes, undrained

1 T. Light Italian Salad Dressing

1 T. fat free cream cheese

¼ t. dried basil

1 oz whole wheat spaghetti noodles, dry

1 oz fresh Parmesan cheese

1. Sautee onions in a large skillet on medium heat until they begin to be translucent. Add meat and cook until cooked through, stirring frequently. Drain any excess grease from pan.

2. Meanwhile cook spaghetti noodles.

3. Stir in spaghetti sauce and tomatoes. Bring to a boil. Reduce heat to medium-low and simmer 15 minutes. Remove from heat and stir in cream cheese, seasonings and Italian salad dressing. Serve hot over cooked spaghetti squash noodles. Top with parmesan cheese.

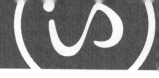

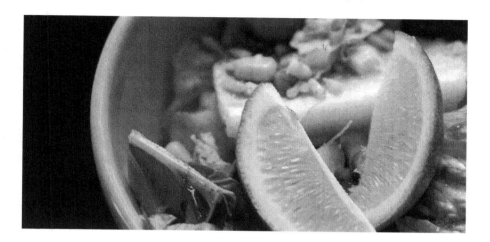

Garlic Lime Chicken Salad

3 T. low sodium soy sauce

1 T. lime juice

2 t. Worcestershire sauce

1 clove garlic

½ t. dry mustard

½ t. pepper

4 oz Chicken breast

1-2 cups romaine lettuce, chopped

Green onion, diced

¼ c. Corn

5 Cherry tomatoes, halved

¼ c. Peas

1 stick celery, diced

1 oz feta cheese

⅓ c. brown rice

1. Combine the first six ingredients for your sauce. Reserve 1 T. of the sauce for salad dressing.

2. Marinate chicken in the rest of the sauce for 15-30 minutes and grill.

3. Meanwhile assemble salad ingredients. Toss salad with rice, veggies, cheese and reserved sauce. Top with chicken.

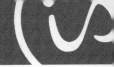

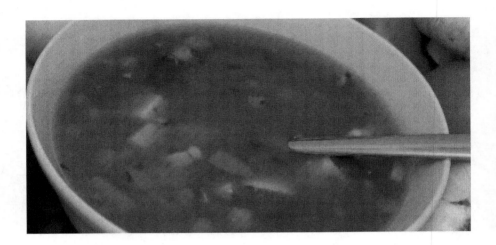

Vegetable, Beef and Barley Stew

4 oz extra lean ground beef

¼ can (14.5 oz) stewed tomatoes, undrained, cut up

¼ (14 oz) can beef broth

¼ can (8 oz) no salt added tomato sauce

1 c. frozen mixed veggies

3 T. quick cooking barley

⅓ avocado

1. *Brown ground beef and drain. In saucepan combine all ingredients and heat to boiling. Reduce heat to medium. Cover and cook 10-15 minutes, stirring occasionally until vegetables and barley are tender. Top with avocado.*

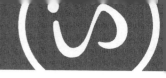

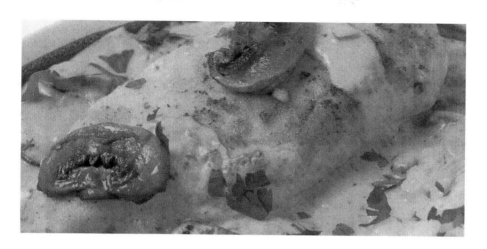

Creamy Crock Pot Chicken

3 oz Chicken breast

½ can cream of chicken soup

4 Sliced mushrooms

½ garlic cloves, pressed

¼ t. Worcestershire sauce

¼ t. lemon juice

1 slice turkey bacon, cooked
   and crumbled

¼ t. vinegar

1 oz cheddar cheese

½ c. white rice, prepared

1. *Combine all ingredients except cheese, rice and chicken breast in a mixing bowl and mix well.*

2. *Put chicken into a crock pot. Cover with soup mixture.*

3. *Cook on low 4-6 hours or until cooked through.*

4. *While still hot top with shredded cheese and allow to melt. Serve with ½ c. white rice and steamed veggies.*

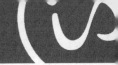

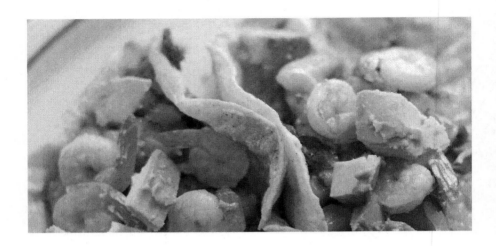

Honey Lime Shrimp Tacos

1 Corn Tortilla

4 oz Shrimp

½ Mango

1-2 cups chopped cabbage

Cilantro

Red Onion

1 t. Honey

1 lime

¼ Avocado

1 t. coconut oil

1. *Warm your pan over medium heat and toast corn tortilla until it's slightly crispy.*

2. *Add 1 t. coconut oil to the pan and cook shrimp for 2-3 minutes.*

3. *Drizzle honey and squeeze the juice of half a lime onto the shrimp. Cook for another 3-4 minutes or until cooked through.*

4. *Meanwhile, dice mango and red onion and chop cilantro.*

5. *Assemble tacos drizzling the sauce over the shrimp. Top with cabbage, mango, onion and avocado.*

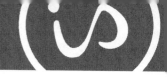

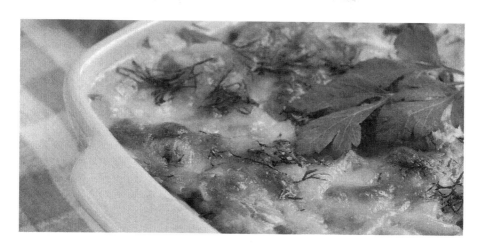

English Muffin Casserole

1 turkey sausage

1 whole wheat english muffin

½ oz low fat mozzarella cheese, shredded

½ oz low fat cheddar cheese, shredded

1 T. chopped onion

1 T. chopped bell pepper

½ c. egg beaters

¼ c. milk

Salt and pepper to taste

1 slice turkey bacon

1. Cook sausage according to package directions. Cool slightly and cut into slices.

2. Cut English muffin into 1 inch cubes and put in greased single serving baking dish.

3. Layer with sausage, cheese, onion and bell pepper.

4. In a separate bowl combine eggs, milk, salt and pepper. Pour over the sausage and cheese mixture.

5. Top with crumbled bacon. Cover and refrigerate overnight.

6. Remove from the fridge 30 minutes prior to baking. Uncover and bake at 350 degrees for about 30 minutes or until a toothpick inserted in the center comes out clean. Let stand for 5 minutes before eating.

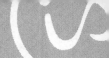

MEN UNDER 250 lbs

If you're a man currently weighing under 250 lbs, here is everything you need to put IdealPlan into action today! This meal plan is targeted to your gender and body weight range to help you reach your goals faster.

Remember: Make sure to use the recipes and food lists that go with your specific meal plan. The calorie amounts and portions of each macronutrient (carbs, proteins and fats) are slightly different for each weight/gender category.

This program is simple on purpose: we've done all the math for you, giving you the calorie amount and balance of carbs, proteins and fats that are generally ideal for fat loss for your weight range. We've also selected foods that fit great with this template, but if you prefer to use your own comparable substitutions, that's fine too!

Because every body is different and physical activity levels vary from person to person, you can use the checkin points at the end of Phase 1 and Phase 2 (see FAQ) to adjust the plan according to your results

Bookmark the first 5 pages for daily reference!

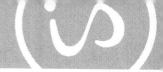
Five-Meal Template

Breakfast Smoothie

1 scoop IdealShake

1 serving fruit (see fruit list)

1 Protein B List Serving

1 c. any milk (see milk list)

Or: choose from the recipes
that follow

Mid-Morning Snack

1 IdealBar

15 almonds

Or: 1 Protein A List Option

1 Carb B List Option

15 almonds

Lunch Smoothie

1 scoop IdealShake

1 Carb D List serving

1 Fat C List serving

1 Protein B List serving

1 c. any milk

Or: choose from the recipes
that follow

Mid-Afternoon Snack

1 Protein B List Serving

1 Carb E List Serving

Or: choose from the recipes
that follow

Optional: 1 IdealBoost stick pack

Dinner:

1 serving any lean meat - 4-6 oz
(approx size of your palm)

1 Fat D List serving

1 Carb F List serving Unlimited
vegetables*

Or: choose from the recipes
that follow

Approximate daily calories: **1800**

40% carbs | 30% proteins | 30% fats

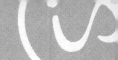

Food Lists

Milk Options:
Almond Milk

Soy Milk

Skim Milk

Low fat Milk

Unsweetened Coconut Milk

Coconut Water

Rice Milk

Fruit Servings:
1 banana

1 apple

1 orange

1 peach

1 pear

1 mango

2 tangerines

2 apricots

2 kiwis

1 c. berries/cherries/pineapple

1 ½ c. any melon (watermelon, cantaloupe, honeydew, etc)

1 ½ c. grapes

1 c. any fruit juice/veggie juice

Or: Any fruit for approx 100 calories

Carb B List (Snack Ideas):
1 flavored rice cakes

½ c. low sugar cereal (e.g., Plain cheerios, Rice Chex, Wheaties, etc)

1 low fat graham crackers

½ serving Whole Wheat Crackers

½ serving fruit (see fruit list)

½ serving pop chips/baked chips

Or: Any low fat carb for approx 50 calories

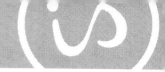

Carb D List (Shake Add-Ins):

½ c. oats

2 T. chia seeds

1 fruit serving (see fruit list)

4 T. PB2 peanut butter powder

2 T. Honey/Agave/Real Maple Syrup

½ c. Plain Cheerios stirred in (or other low sugar cereal)

1 flavored yogurt

2 low fat graham crackers

Or: Any low fat carb for approx 150 calories

Carb E List (Snack Ideas):

2 flavored rice cakes

1 c. low sugar cereal (e.g., Plain cheerios, Rice Chex, Wheaties, etc)

2 low fat graham crackers

1 serving whole wheat crackers

1 serving fruit

1 slice whole wheat bread

3 c. Air Popped Popcorn

1 serving Popped/baked chips

Or: Any low fat carb for approx 100 calories

Carb F List (Dinner Options):

¾ c. brown/white rice

¾ c. couscous

¾ c. quinoa

¾ c. whole wheat pasta

1 medium sweet/red/white potato

1 whole wheat tortilla

3 corn tortillas

1 ½ slices whole wheat bread

1 ½ servings fruit (see fruit list)

Or: Any low fat carb for approx 150 calories

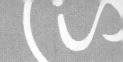

Protein A Servings (Shake Add-Ins/Snack Options):

½ c. low fat cottage cheese

¾ c. plain fat free Greek yogurt

½ scoop whey protein

1 80-100 calorie flavored Greek yogurt (e.g., Chobani)

¾ c. liquid egg whites (can be added to shakes to make them smooth and creamy)

1 egg (hard boiled are easily transportable)

1 oz beef jerky

3 oz Turkey slices

1 low fat string cheese

1 servings tuna

Or: Any protein for approx 100 calories

Protein B Servings (Shake Add-Ins/Snack Options):

¾ c. low fat cottage cheese

1 c. plain fat free Greek yogurt

1 scoop whey protein

150 calorie flavored Greek yogurt (e.g., Chobani)

1 c. liquid egg whites (can be added to shakes to make them smooth and creamy)

2 eggs (hard boiled are easily transportable)

2 oz beef jerky

5 oz Turkey slices

2 low fat string cheese

1 ½ servings tuna

Or: Any protein for approx 150 calories

Fat C List (Shake Add-Ins):

2 T. peanut butter

¾ avocado

4 T. flax seed

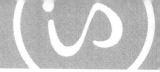

1 ½ T. coconut oil

6 T. coconut flakes

1 ½ oz dark chocolate

Or: Any low sugar fat for approx 200 calories

Fat D List (Dinner Options):

2 oz cheese

2 T. any nuts/seeds/nut butter

½ c. feta cheese

2 T. any oil (coconut, extra virgin olive oil, grapeseed oil, etc)

2 T. any salad dressing

⅓ avocado

Or: Any low sugar fat for approx 200 calories

Freebie Shake Add-Ins:

2 T. Sugar free fat free pudding powder

1 T. Cocoa Powder

Any Extracts - vanilla, coconut, almond, maple, orange, etc

Sugar Free Syrups (e.g., Torani and DaVinci)

¼ t. Crystal Light mix

Any Vegetables*

---

*Vegetable Cheat Sheet

Fibrous veggies are allowed with any meal in any amount (e.g., asparagus, broccoli, Brussels sprouts, cabbage, cauliflower, celery, okra, cucumber, eggplant, collard greens, tomato, leek, lettuce, any mushroom, green onion, onion, bell pepper, radish, snow peas, spinach, zucchini, fennel, green beans, pickles).

Carrots, peas and squash are not "free" veggies but can be enjoyed occasionally.

Corn and potatoes are counted as grains/carbs in the meal plan.

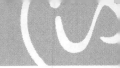

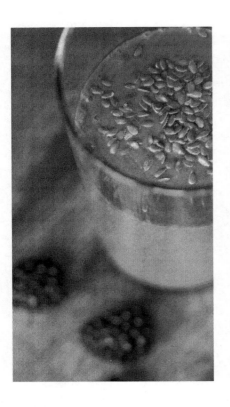

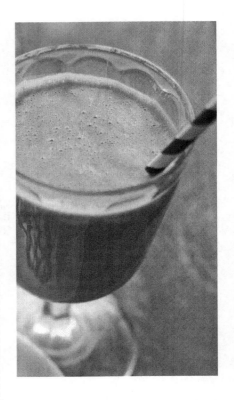

Black Berry Boost

1 scoop Vanilla IdealShake

1 c. unsweetened almond milk

1 c. fresh blackberries

½ c. low fat cottage cheese

½ c. liquid egg whites

Ice Cubes

Chocolate Banana

1 scoop Chocolate IdealShake

1 c. unsweetened almond milk

1 banana

1 c. plain fat free Greek yogurt

Ice Cubes

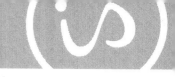

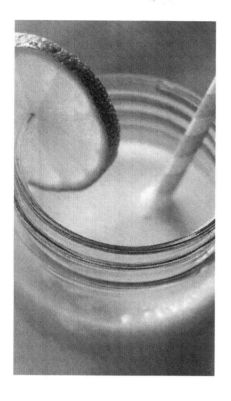

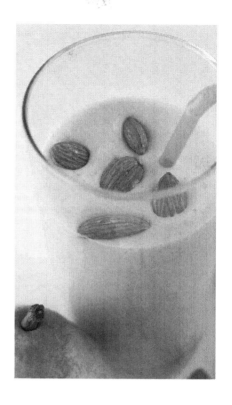

Key Lime Pie

1 scoop Vanilla IdealShake

1 unsweetened almond milk

1 T. lime juice

1 low fat graham cracker *

¾ c. low fat cottage cheese

Ice Cubes

Graham cracker subs for the fruit in your breakfast shake

Almond Pear Spice

1 scoop Vanilla IdealShake

¾ c. unsweetened almond milk

½ c. liquid egg whites

½ c. low fat cottage cheese

½ banana

½ pear

1 t. cinnamon

1 t. almond extract

Ice Cubes

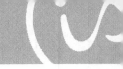

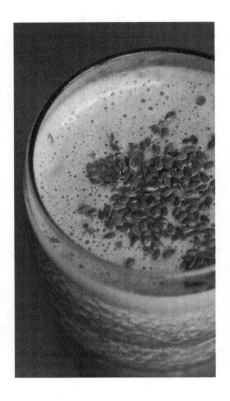

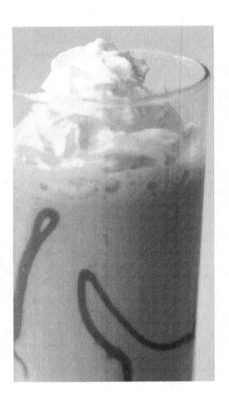

Tropical Greens

1 scoop Vanilla IdealShake

1 c. coconut water

1 c. plain fat free Greek yogurt

½ c. strawberries

½ c. pineapple

1 c. spinach

Ice Cubes

Salted Caramel Pumpkin Latte

1 scoop Mocha or Vanilla IdealShake

½ c. coffee, cooled

½ c. unswt almond milk

¾ c. low fat cottage cheese

2 T. canned pumpkin

½ banana

1-2 T. sugar free Torani Salted Caramel Syrup

Pinch of sea salt

Ice Cubes

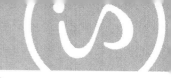

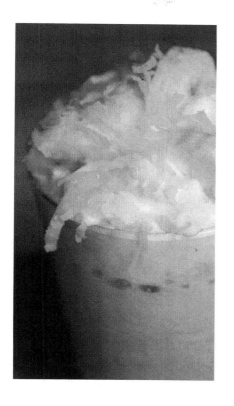

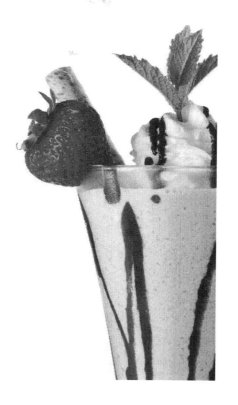

Banana Coconut Coffee

1 scoop Mocha IdealShake

½ c. unswt coconut milk

½ c. liquid egg whites

1 banana

1 container Coconut Dannon Light n
Fit Greek Yogurt

1-2 T. sugar free Torani Coconut Syrup

Ice Cubes

Triple Chocolate Berry

1 scoop Chocolate IdealShake

1 c. Hood Carb Countdown Chocolate
Milk

¾ c. frozen strawberries

¾ c. low fat cottage cheese

2 T. sugar free chocolate pudding
powder

Ice Cubes

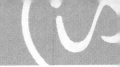

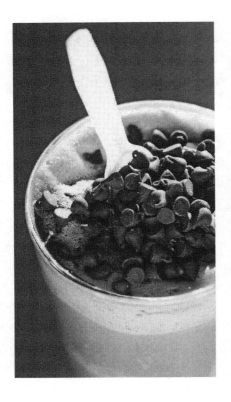

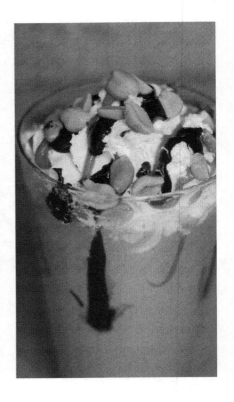

Minty Mocha

1 scoop Mocha IdealShake

¼ c. unsweetened almond milk or cooled coffee

1 c. liquid egg whites

½ t. peppermint extract

Ice Cubes

Have one piece of fruit on the side.

Candybar

1 scoop Chocolate IdealShake

1 c. unsweetened almond milk

¾ c. low fat cottage cheese

2 T. PB2 peanut butter powder (in place of fruit in template)

1 t. cocoa powder

2 t. sugar free caramel syrup

Ice Cubes

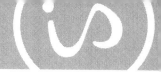

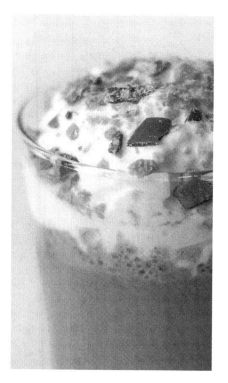

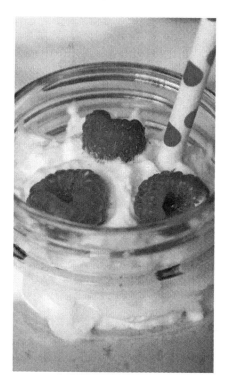

The Butter-Finger

1 scoop Chocolate IdealShake

1 c. Hood Carb Countdown chocolate
milk

2 T. peanut butter

¾ c. low fat cottage cheese

1 T. sugar free fat free butterscotch
pudding powder

½ c. oats

½ T. unsweetened cocoa

Sweetener to taste

Ice Cubes

Raspberry Cheesecake

1 scoop Vanilla IdealShake

1 c. unsweetened almond milk

1 c. frozen/fresh raspberries

1 graham cracker sheet

1 oz dark chocolate*

¾ c. low fat cottage cheese

Ice cubes

*Dark chocolate can be sprinkled over
the top or blended in*

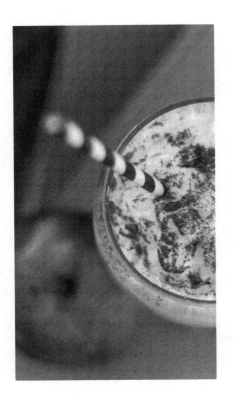

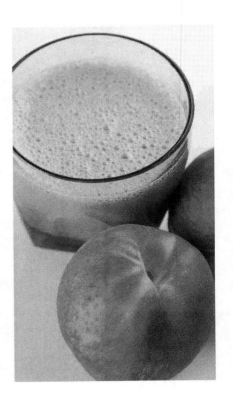

Apple Pie A La Mode

1 scoop vanilla IdealShake

1 c. unsweetened almond milk

½ c. unsweetened applesauce

½ c. vanilla Greek yogurt

½ c. low fat cottage cheese

½ t. apple pie spice

¼ oats*

2 T. peanut butter

Ice Cubes

Blend most of the oats into the shake but save 1-2 T to sprinkle the oats over the top of the shake

Peachy Greens

1 scoop Vanilla IdealShake

1 c. orange juice

½ c. liquid egg whites

1 peach, pitted

¾ avocado

½ c. plain fat free Greek yogurt

1 c. spinach

Ice cubes

146

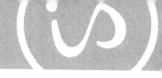

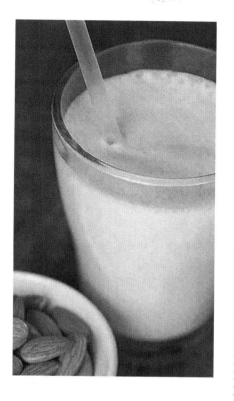

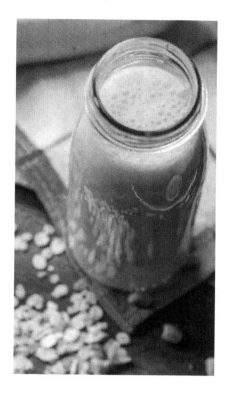

Honey Nut

1 scoop Vanilla IdealShake

1 c. unsweetened almond milk

⅓ c. liquid egg whites

3 T. PB2 peanut butter powder

1 T. honey

2 T. Almond butter

½ c. low fat cottage cheese

Ice Cubes

Peanut Butter Cookie

1 scoop Chocolate or Vanilla
IdealShake

1 c. unswt almond milk

1 c. plain greek yogurt

½ c. oats

2 T. peanut butter

Sweetener, if desired

Ice Cubes

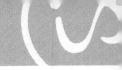

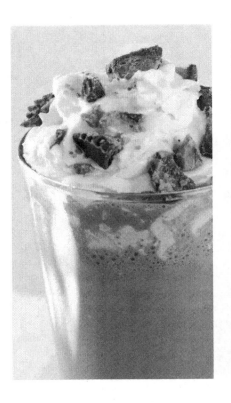

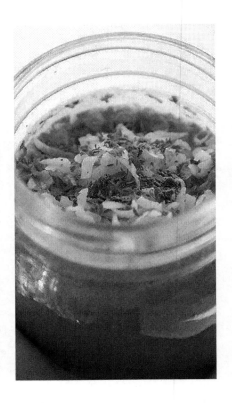

Chocolate Peanut Butter Cup

1 scoop Chocolate IdealShake

1 c. unswt almond milk

¾ c. low fat cottage cheese

3 T. PB2 peanut butter powder

¼ c. oats

2 T. Peanut butter

Ice Cubes

Almond Delight

1 scoop Chocolate IdealShake

1 scoop Chocolate IdealShake

1 c. dark chocolate almond milk

¾ c. low fat cottage cheese

¼ c. oats

1 T. chia seeds

¼ c. part skim ricotta

1 T. coconut flakes, sprinkled over the top

12 g. slivered almonds, sprinkled over the top

Ice Cubes

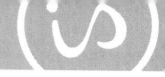

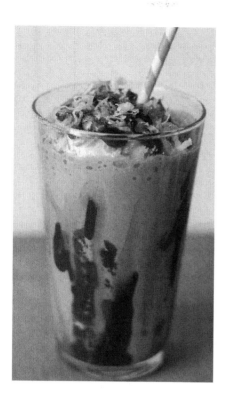

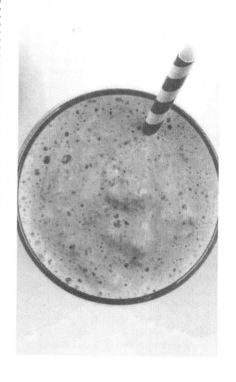

Caramel Coconut Cookie

1 scoop Chocolate IdealShake

1 c. unswt coconut milk

¾ c. low fat cottage cheese

¼ t. coconut extract

2 T. sugar free caramel syrup ice cream

1 T. sugar free chocolate syrup ice cream

2 T. oats

1 T. coconut oil, melted*

1 T. coconut flakes

Ice Cubes

Melt the coconut oil and then drizzle slowly into shake while blender is mixing to prevent clumping.

Berries n Cream

1 scoop Strawberry IdealShake

1 c. unswt almond milk

1 c. fat free plain greek yogurt

½ c. frozen raspberries

½ c. frozen strawberries

2 T. sugar free french vanilla creamer

1 T. fat free sugar free vanilla pudding mix

¼ c. oats

2 T. flax seeds

⅓ avocado

Ice Cubes

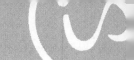

Optional:
1 IdealBoost Stick Pack drink on the side with your snack!

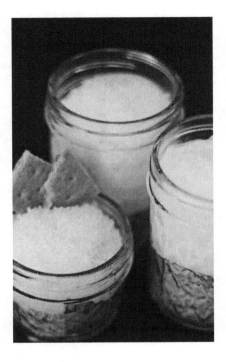

Coconut Cream Pie

1 container Coconut Chobani Greek yogurt

2 low fat graham cracker, crumbled

Stir graham cracker crumbs into yogurt.

Fruit and Eggs

1 ½ c. grapes

2 hardboiled eggs

Berries 'n' Cream

1 c. low fat cottage cheese

1 c. strawberries

Cinnamon and stevia, to taste

Stir berries into cottage cheese and top with cinnamon and stevia

Tuna "Sandwich"

3 oz tuna

1 hard boiled egg

½ T. light mayo

2 lightly salted rice cakes

Mix tuna and mayo and spread over the rice cake.

Have egg on the side or mix into the tuna salad.

Easy Cheesecake

½ c. plain fat free Greek yogurt

½ c. low fat cottage cheese

2 T. sugar free cheesecake pudding powder

1 c. plain cheerios

Sautee the cheerios on a pan over medium heat with spray butter and salt. Stir often. When they're lightly toasted cool in a bowl.

Stir stevia and pudding powder into the Greek yogurt.

Top the yogurt with the cheerios and enjoy!

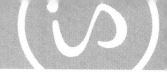

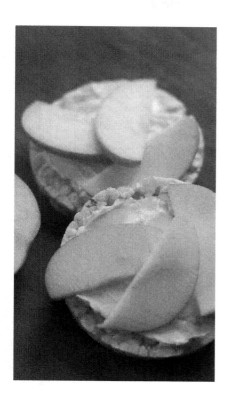

Fruit and Jerky

1 banana

2 oz beef jerky

·····································

Cheesy Rice Cake Snack

2 cheddar rice cakes

¾ c. low fat cottage cheese

Top the rice cake with cottage cheese

·····································

Cheese and Crackers

1 serving whole wheat crackers

2 string cheese sticks

·····································

Turkey Sandwich

2 slices low carb 45 calorie Sara Lee
  bread

4 oz turkey

½ T. light mayo

Lettuce, tomato, onion

*Make a turkey sandwich and add
lettuce tomato and onion*

Apple Swiss Rice Cakes

2 wedges light Laughing Cow cheese

⅓ c. low fat cottage cheese

1 small granny smith apple, thinly
  sliced

2 lightly salted rice cakes

*Spread the cheese over the rice cake
and top with apple slices*

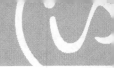

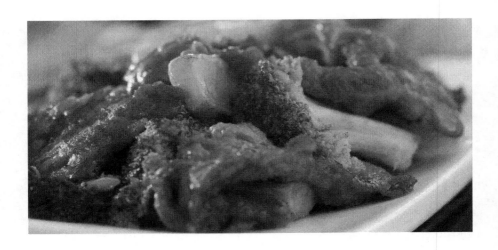

Beef and Broccoli Stir Fry

5 oz lean beef such as Top Sirloin, Flank or London Broil, sliced into thin slices

½ t. minced garlic

¼ t. ginger

½ T. light soy sauce

1 c. broccoli

½ T. coconut oil

2 T. water

6 T. beef broth / T. cornstarch

¼ c. bean sprouts, optional

2 T. peanuts, chopped

¾ c. brown rice, cooked

1. Combine beef, garlic, ginger and soy sauce in a bowl and let stand.

2. Wash broccoli thoroughly and cut into florets.

3. Heat 1 t. oil in a nonstick skillet over high heat, add broccoli and stir fry for 2 minutes. Add water and stir until the water evaporates. Move broccoli to a separate bowl.

4. Heat remaining 2 t. oil, and add beef mixture. Stir fry for 3 minutes. Stir together broth and cornstarch, add to meat and stir fry until sauce is thickened, about 3 more minutes.

5. Add broccoli and bean sprouts, then cook, stirring, until heated through, about 2 more minutes.

6. Top with 2 T. chopped peanuts, spread over % c. brown rice and enjoy!

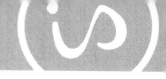

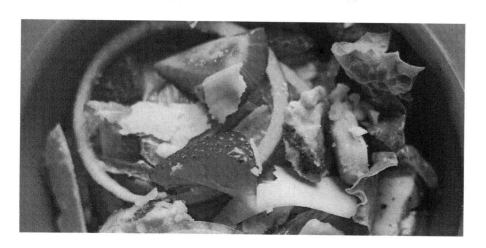

Maple Chicken Salad

Salad:

5 oz chicken, cooked and cut into strips

Romaine Lettuce

Red onion, thinly sliced

5 large strawberries

1 oz swiss cheese, shredded

2 slices turkey bacon, cooked and crumbled

¾ c. quinoa, cooked

Dressing:

½ T. extra virgin olive oil

1 T. vinegar

½ T. light mayo

½ T. sugar free maple syrup

4 pecans, chopped, optional

Stevia to taste, if needed

1. *Combine dressing ingredients and allow to sit for 15-30 minutes in the fridge.*

2. *Meanwhile combine salad ingredients.*

3. *Toss salad in dressing and enjoy!*

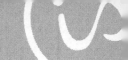

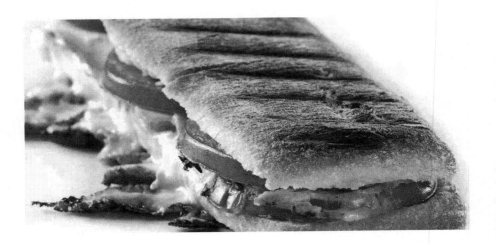

Balsamic Chicken Panini

6 oz chicken

½ c. Balsamic Vinegar

Whole bell pepper, thinly sliced

Sweet onion, thinly sliced

⅓ avocado, sliced

1 oz provolone cheese, sliced

1 Small focaccia roll (approx 150 calories)

1. Slice chicken breast in half so that it's cut thinly. Sautee in ¼ c. vinegar until cooked through.

2. Place chicken in a separate bowl. Sautee peppers and onion in ¼ c. vinegar until soft and cooked through.

3. Spray both sides of the sandwich thin with spray butter and assemble sandwich with chicken, veggies, avocado and cheese.

4. Grill the sandwich on an indoor grill (ie George Foreman) or on the stove in a pan over medium heat.

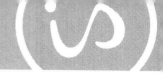

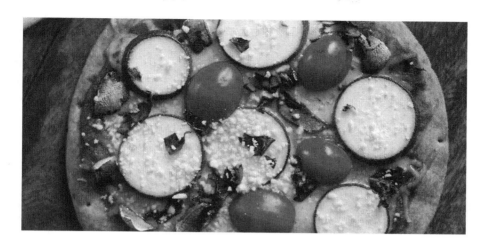

Low Carb Grilled Chicken Pizza

½ zucchini, thinly sliced

2 mushrooms, sliced

1 pitas or whole wheat tortillas (approx 150 calories)

3-4 T. tomato basil pizza sauce

3 oz low fat mozzarella cheese

4 cherry tomatoes

5 oz chicken, cooked and sliced

1 T. fresh basil, chopped

1. Preheat oven to 180 degrees.

2. Grill or roast zucchini and mushrooms until desired tenderness.* Transfer to a plate.

3. Place tortillas on a baking tray lined with foil. Spread sauce over tortillas and sprinkle with ½ oz of cheese. Top with grilled veggies, tomatoes and chicken. Top with remaining cheese.

4. Bake for 12-15 minutes or until tortilla is crisp and cheese is melted. Sprinkle with basil and serve with a side salad.

*To grill veggies preheat gas grill over medium heat. Spray the veggies with spray butter or cooking spray and lightly salt them. Cook over low-med heat for approx 5-8 minutes or until desired tenderness is reached. To roast veggies preheat oven to 400 degrees and bake on a baking sheet for approx 20-25 minute or until desired tenderness is reached. Then let oven cool before baking pizza.

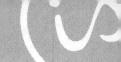

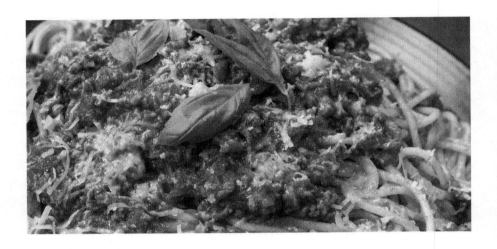

Creamy Bolognese over Spaghetti

¼ yellow onion, chopped

½ clove garlic

5 oz extra lean ground beef

½ c. premade spaghetti sauce

¼ can (14 oz) diced tomatoes, undrained

1 T. Light Italian Salad Dressing

1 T. fat free cream cheese

¼ t. dried basil

½ oz whole wheat spaghetti noodles, dry

1 oz fresh Parmesan cheese

1. *Sautee onions in a large skillet on medium heat until begin to be translucent. Add meat and cook until cooked through, stirring frequently. Drain any excess grease from pan.*

2. *Meanwhile cook spaghetti noodles.*

3. *Stir in spaghetti sauce and tomatoes. Bring to a boil. Reduce heat to medium-low and simmer 15 minutes. Remove from heat and stir in cream cheese, seasonings and Italian salad dressing. Serve hot over cooked spaghetti squash noodles. Top with parmesan*

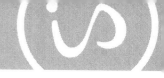

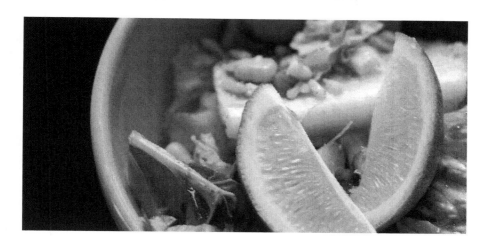

Garlic Lime Chicken Salad

3 T. low sodium soy sauce

1 T. lime juice

2 t. Worcestershire sauce

1 clove garlic

½ t. dry mustard

½ t. pepper

6 oz Chicken breast

1-2 cups romaine lettuce, chopped

Green onion, diced

¼ c. Corn

5 Cherry tomatoes, halved

¼ c. Peas

1 stick celery, diced

2 oz feta cheese

¾ c. brown rice

1. *Combine the first six ingredients for your sauce. Reserve 1 T. of the sauce for salad dressing.*

2. *Marinate chicken in the rest of the sauce for 15-30 minutes and grill.*

3. *Meanwhile assemble salad ingredients. Toss salad with rice, veggies, cheese and reserved sauce. Top with chicken.*

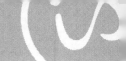

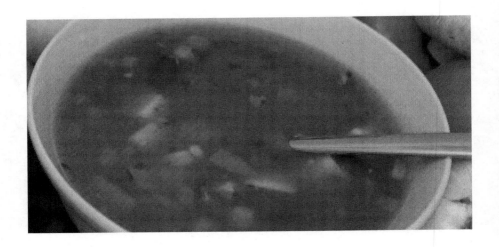

Vegetable, Beef and Barley Stew

7 oz extra lean ground beef

¼ can (14.5 oz) stewed tomatoes, undrained, cut up

¼ (14 oz) can beef broth

¼ can (8 oz) no salt added tomato sauce

1 c. frozen mixed veggies

5 T. quick cooking barley

½ avocado, diced

1. *Brown ground beef and drain. In saucepan combine all ingredients and heat to boiling. Reduce heat to medium. Cover and cook 10-15 minutes, stirring occasionally until vegetables and barley are tender. Top with avocado.*

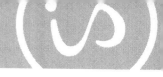

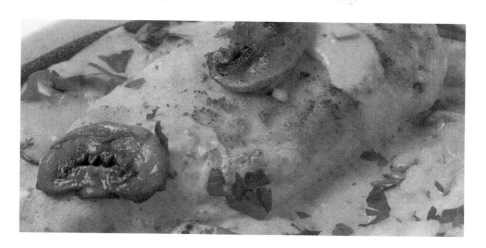

Creamy Crock Pot Chicken

5 oz Chicken breast

½ can cream of chicken soup

4 Sliced mushrooms

½ garlic cloves, pressed

¼ t. Worcestershire sauce

¼ t. lemon juice

1 slice turkey bacon, cooked and
  crumbled

¼ t. vinegar

2 oz cheddar cheese

¾ c. white rice, prepared

1. *Combine all ingredients except cheese, rice and chicken breast in a mixing bowl and mix well.*

2. *Put chicken into a crock pot. Cover with soup mixture.*

3. *Cook on low 4-6 hours or until cooked through.*

4. *While still hot top with shredded cheese and allow to melt. Serve with ½ c. white rice and steamed veggies.*

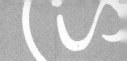

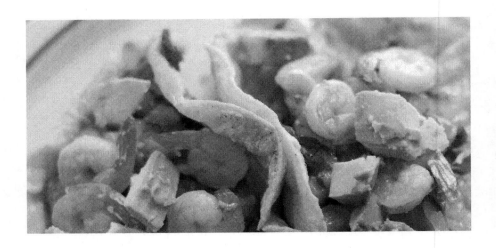

Honey Lime Shrimp Tacos

2 Corn Tortilla

8 oz Shrimp

½ Mango

1-2 c. chopped cabbage

Cilantro

Red Onion

1 t. Honey

1 lime

½ Avocado

1 t. coconut oil

1. Warm your pan over medium heat and toast corn tortilla until it's slightly crispy.

2. Add 1 t. coconut oil to the pan and cook shrimp for 2-3 minutes.

3. Drizzle honey and squeeze the juice of half a lime onto the shrimp. Cook for another 3-4 minutes or until cooked through.

4. Meanwhile, dice mango and red onion and chop cilantro.

5. Assemble tacos drizzling the sauce over the shrimp. Top with cabbage, mango, onion and avocado.

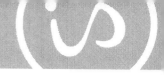

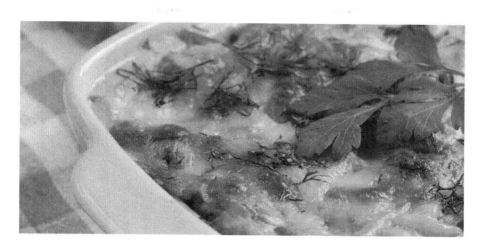

English Muffin Casserole

1 turkey sausage

1½ whole wheat English muffins

1 oz low fat mozzarella cheese, shredded

1 oz low fat cheddar cheese, shredded

1 T. chopped onion

1 T. chopped bell pepper

2 eggs

¼ c. egg beaters

¼ c. milk

Salt and pepper to taste

1 slice turkey bacon

1. Cook sausage according to package directions. Cool slightly and cut into slices.

2. Cut English muffin into 1 inch cubes and put in greased single serving baking dish.

3. Layer with sausage, cheese, onion and bell pepper.

4. In a separate bowl combine eggs, milk, salt and pepper. Pour over the sausage and cheese mixture.

5. Top with crumbled bacon. Cover and refrigerate overnight.

6. Remove from the fridge 30 minutes prior to baking. Uncover and bake at 350 degrees for about 30 minutes or until a toothpick inserted in the center comes out clean. Let stand for 5 minutes before eating.

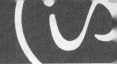

MEN OVER 250 lbs

If you're a man currently weighing over 250 lbs, here is everything you need to put IdealPlan into action today! This meal plan is targeted to your gender and body weight range to help you reach your goals faster.

Remember: Make sure to use the recipes and food lists that go with your specific meal plan. The calorie amounts and portions of each macronutrient (carbs, proteins and fats) are slightly different for each weight/gender category.

This program is simple on purpose: we've done all the math for you, giving you the calorie amount and balance of carbs, proteins and fats that are generally ideal for fat loss for your weight range. We've also selected foods that fit great with this template, but if you prefer to use your own comparable substitutions, that's fine too!

Because every body is different and physical activity levels vary from person to person, you can use the checkin points at the end of Phase 1 and Phase 2 (see FAQ) to adjust the plan according to your results

Bookmark the first 4 pages for daily reference!

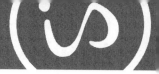

Five-Meal Template

Breakfast Smoothie

1 scoop IdealShake

1 large serving fruit (see fruit list)

1 Carb A serving

1 Protein B Serving

1 c. any milk (see milk list)

Or: choose from the recipes that follow

Mid-Morning Snack

1 IdealBar

15 almonds

Or: 1 Protein A List Option

1 Carb B List Option

15 almonds

Lunch Smoothie

1 scoop IdealShake

1 Carb D List serving

1 Fat C List serving

1 Protein B List serving

1 c. any milk

Or: choose from the recipes that follow

Mid-Afternoon Snack

1 Protein B List Serving

1 Carb E List Serving

Optional: 1 IdealBoost stick pack

Or: choose from the recipes that follow

Dinner

1 ½ servings any lean meat (7-8 oz -

approx size of palm of hand times 1 ½)

1 Fat D List serving

1 Carb G List serving

Unlimited vegetables*

Or: choose from the recipes that follow

Approximate daily calories: **2400**

40% carbs | 30% proteins | 30% fats

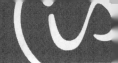

Food Lists

Milk Options:
Almond Milk

Soy Milk

Skim Milk

Low fat Milk

Unsweetened Coconut Milk

Coconut Water

Rice Milk

Fruit Servings:
1 banana

1 apple

1 orange

1 peach

1 pear

1 mango

2 tangerines

2 apricots

2 kiwis

1 c. berries/cherries/pineapple

1 ½ c. any melon (watermelon, cantaloupe, honeydew, etc)

1 ½ c. grapes

1 c. any fruit juice/veggie juice

Or: Any fruit for approx 100 calories

Carb A Options (Shake Add-Ins):
¼ c. oats

1 T. chia seeds

½ fruit serving (see fruit list)

2 T. PB2 peanut butter powder

1 T. Honey/Agave/Real Maple Syrup

¼ c. Plain cheerios (stirred in)

1 light yogurt

1 low fat graham cracker

Or: Any low fat carb for approx 75 calories

Carb B List (Small Snacks):
1 flavored rice cake

½ c. low sugar cereal (Plain Cheerios, Rice Chex, Wheaties, etc)

1 low fat graham cracker

½ serving whole wheat crackers

½ serving pop chips/baked chips

½ serving fruit (see fruit list)

Or: Any low fat carb for approx 50 calories

Carb D List (Shake Add-Ins):
½ c. oats

2 T. chia seeds

1 fruit serving (see fruit list)

4 T. PB2 peanut butter powder

2 T. Honey/Agave/Real Maple Syrup

½ c. Plain Cheerios stirred in (or other low sugar cereal)

1 flavored yogurt

2 low fat graham crackers

Or: Any low fat carb for approx 150 calories

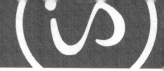

Carb E List (Snack Ideas):

2 flavored rice cakes

1 c. low sugar cereal (Plain cheerios, Rice Chex, Wheaties, etc)

2 low fat graham crackers

1 serving Whole Wheat Crackers

1 serving fruit

1 slice Whole wheat bread

3 c. Air Popped Popcorn

1 serving Popped/baked chips

Or: Any low fat carb for approx 100 calories

Carb G List (Dinner Options):

1 c. brown/white rice

1 c. couscous

1 c. quinoa

1 c. whole wheat pasta

1 large sweet/red/white potato

2 small whole wheat tortillas or 1 large whole wheat tortilla

4 corn tortillas

2 slices Whole Wheat bread

2 servings fruit

Or: Any Low fat Carb for approx 200 calories

Protein A Servings (Shake Add-Ins/Snack Options):

½ c. low fat cottage cheese

¾ c. fat free plain Greek yogurt

½ scoop whey protein

1 80-100 calorie flavored Greek yogurt (e.g., Dannon Light n Fit Greek)

¾ c. liquid egg whites (can be added to shakes to make it smooth and creamy)

1 egg (hard boiled is easily transportable)

1 oz beef jerky

3 oz turkey slices

1 low fat string cheese

1 serving tuna

Or: Any protein for approx 100 calories

Protein B Servings (Shake Add-Ins/Snack Options):

¾ c. low fat cottage cheese

1 c. plain fat free Greek yogurt

1 scoop whey protein

150 calorie flavored Greek yogurt (e.g., Chobani)

1 c. liquid egg whites (can be added to shakes to make them smooth and creamy)

2 eggs (hard boiled are easily transportable)

2 oz beef jerky

5 oz Turkey slices

2 low fat string cheese

1 ½ servings tuna

Or: Any protein for approx 150 calories

Fat C List (Shake Add-Ins):

2 T. peanut butter

¾ avocado

4 T. flax seed

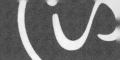

1 ½ T. coconut oil

6 T. coconut flakes

1 ½ oz dark chocolate

Or: Any low sugar fat for approx 200 calories

Fat D List (Dinner Options):

2 oz cheese

2 T. any nuts/seeds/nut butter

½ c. feta cheese

2 T. any oil (coconut, extra virgin olive oil, grapeseed oil, etc)

2 T. any salad dressing

⅔ avocado

Or: Any low sugar fat for approx 200 calories

Freebie Shake Add-In's:

2 T. Sugar free fat free pudding powder

1 T. Cocoa Powder

Any Extracts - vanilla, coconut, almond, maple, orange, etc

Sugar Free Syrups (e.g., Torani and DaVinci)

¼ t. Crystal Light mix

Any Vegetables*

---

*Vegetable Cheat Sheet

Fibrous veggies are allowed with any meal in any amount (e.g., asparagus, broccoli, Brussels sprouts, cabbage, cauliflower, celery, okra, cucumber, eggplant, collard greens, tomato, leek, lettuce, any mushroom, green onion, onion, bell pepper, radish, snow peas, spinach, zucchini, fennel, green beans, pickles).

Carrots, peas and squash are not "free" veggies but can be enjoyed occasionally.

Corn and potatoes are counted as grains/carbs in the meal plan.

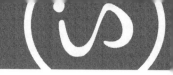

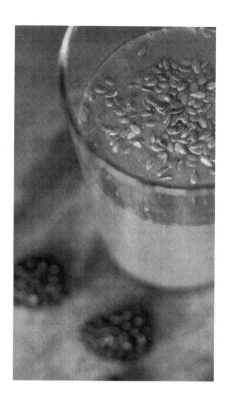

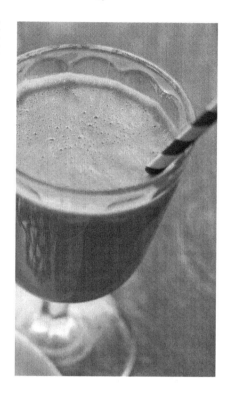

Black Berry Boost

1 scoop Vanilla IdealShake

1 c. unsweetened almond milk

1 c. fresh blackberries

½ c. low fat cottage cheese

⅓ c. liquid egg whites

¼ c. oats

Ice Cubes

Chocolate Banana

1 scoop Chocolate IdealShake

1 c. unsweetened almond milk

1 banana

1 c. plain fat free Greek yogurt

¼ c. plain cheerios*

Ice Cubes

Stir in the cheerios after blending to add some crunch!

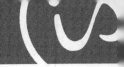

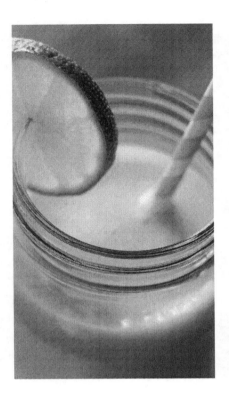

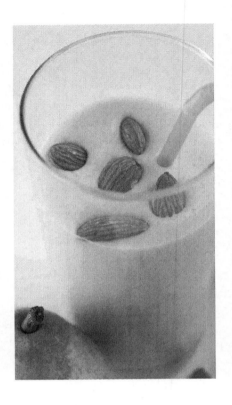

Key Lime Pie

1 scoop Vanilla IdealShake

1 unsweetened almond milk

1 T. lime juice

2 low fat graham crackers*

¾ c. low fat cottage cheese

Ice Cubes

*Graham cracker subs for the fruit
and carb in your breakfast shake. Try
blending one graham cracker into your
shake and crunching the other one up
on top!*

Almond Pear Spice

1 scoop Vanilla IdealShake

¾ c. unsweetened almond milk

⅓ c. liquid egg whites

½ c. low fat cottage cheese

¼ c. oats

½ banana

½ pear

1 t. cinnamon

1 t. almond extract

Ice Cubes

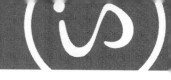

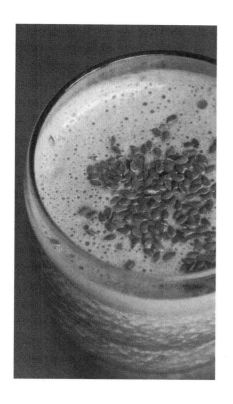

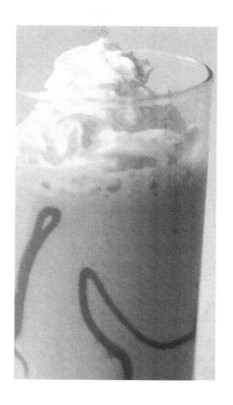

Tropical Greens

1 scoop Vanilla IdealShake

1 c. coconut water

1 c. plain fat free Greek yogurt

1 T. chia seeds

½ c. strawberries

½ c. pineapple

1 c. spinach

Ice Cubes

Salted Caramel Pumpkin Latte

1 scoop Mocha or Vanilla IdealShake

½ cup coffee, cooled

½ c. unswt almond milk

1 T. chia seeds

¾ c. low fat cottage cheese

2 T. canned pumpkin

½ banana

1-2 T. sugar free Torani Salted
   Caramel Syrup

Pinch of sea salt

Ice Cubes

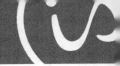

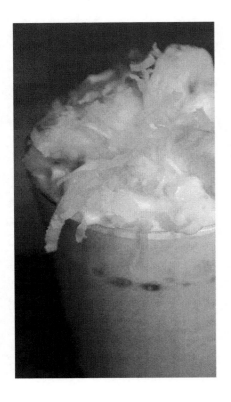

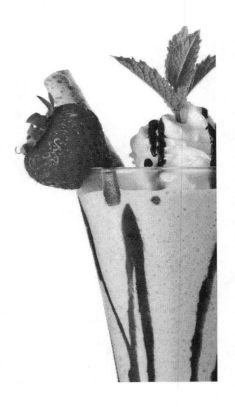

Banana Coconut Coffee

1 scoop Mocha IdealShake

½ c. unswt coconut milk

½ c. liquid egg whites

1 low fat graham cracker

1 banana

1 container Coconut Dannon Light n Fit Greek Yogurt

1-2 T. sugar free Torani Coconut Syrup

Ice Cubes

Triple Chocolate Berry

1 scoop Chocolate IdealShake

1 c. Hood Carb Countdown Chocolate Milk

¾ c. frozen strawberries

¾ c. low fat cottage cheese

2 T. sugar free chocolate pudding powder

Ice Cubes

After blending stir in ¼ c. cheerios and eat with a spoon.

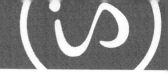

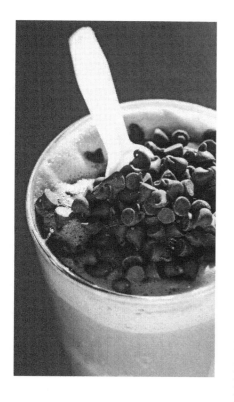

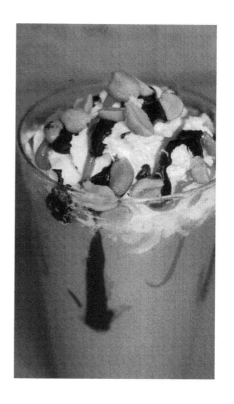

Minty Mocha

1 scoop Mocha IdealShake

¼ c. unsweetened almond milk or
cooled coffee

1 c. liquid egg whites

½ t. peppermint extract

1 T. chia seeds

Ice Cubes

Have one piece of fruit on the side.

Candybar

1 scoop Chocolate IdealShake

1 c. unsweetened almond milk

¾ c. low fat cottage cheese

4 T. PB2 peanut butter powder
(in place of fruit in template)

1 t. cocoa powder

1 ½ T. sugar free caramel syrup

Ice Cubes

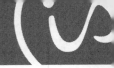

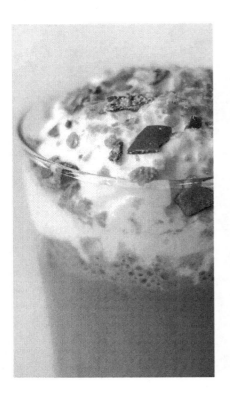

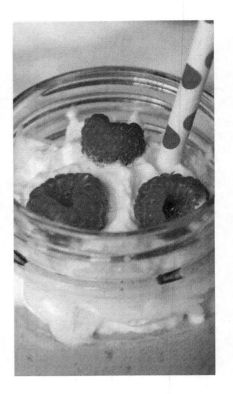

The Butter-Finger

1 scoop Chocolate IdealShake

1 c. Hood Carb Countdown chocolate
milk

2 T. peanut butter

¾ c. low fat cottage cheese

1 T. sugar free fat free butterscotch
pudding powder

½ c. oats

½ T. unsweetened cocoa

Sweetener to taste

Ice Cubes

Raspberry Cheesecake

1 scoop Vanilla IdealShake

1 c. unsweetened almond milk

1 c. frozen/fresh raspberries

1 graham cracker sheet

1 oz dark chocolate*

¾ c. low fat cottage cheese

Ice cubes

*Dark chocolate can be sprinkled over
the top or blended in*

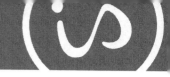

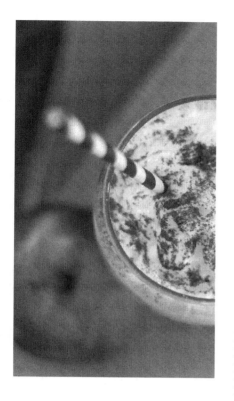

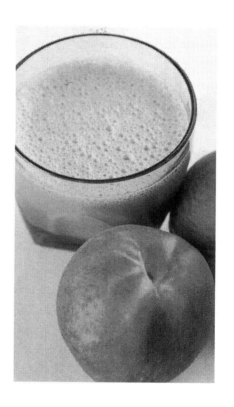

Apple Pie A La Mode

1 scoop vanilla IdealShake

1 c. unsweetened almond milk

½ c. unsweetened applesauce

½ c. vanilla Greek yogurt

½ c. low fat cottage cheese

½ t. apple pie spice

¼ oats*

2 T. peanut butter

Ice Cubes

*Blend most of the oats into the shake
but save 1-2 T to sprinkle the oats
over the top of the shake*

Peachy Greens

1 scoop Vanilla IdealShake

1 c. orange juice

½ c. liquid egg whites

1 peach, pitted

¾ avocado

½ c. plain fat free Greek yogurt

1 c. spinach

Ice cubes

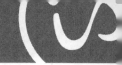

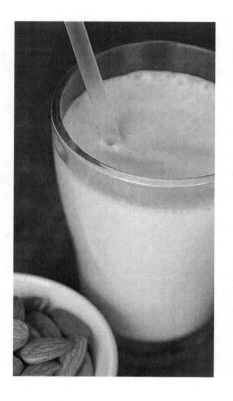

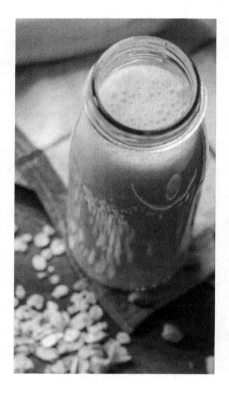

Honey Nut

1 scoop Vanilla IdealShake

1 c. unsweetened almond milk

⅓ c. liquid egg whites

3 T. PB2 peanut butter powder

1 T. honey

2 T. Almond butter

½ c. low fat cottage cheese

Ice Cubes

Peanut Butter Cookie

1 scoop Chocolate or Vanilla
   IdealShake

1 c. unswt almond milk

1 c. plain Greek yogurt

½ c. oats

2 T. peanut butter

Sweetener, if desired

Ice Cubes

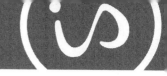

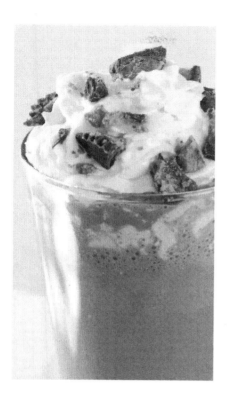

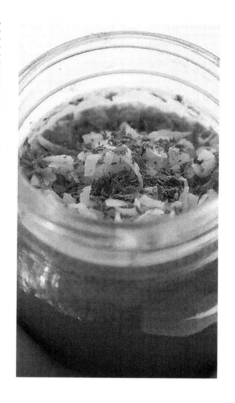

Chocolate Peanut Butter Cup

1 scoop Chocolate IdealShake

1 c. unswt almond milk

¾ c. low fat cottage cheese

3 T. PB2 peanut butter powder

¼ c. oats

2 T. Peanut butter

Ice Cubes

Almond Delight

1 scoop Chocolate IdealShake

1 c. dark chocolate almond milk

¾ c. low fat cottage cheese

¼ c. oats

1 T. chia seeds

¼ c. part skim ricotta

1 T. coconut flakes, sprinkled over
the top

12 g. slivered almonds, sprinkled over
the top

Ice Cubes

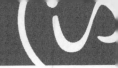

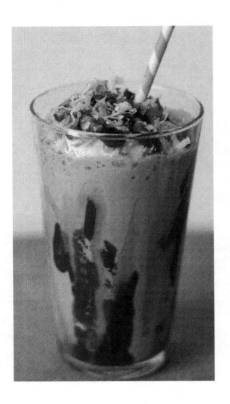

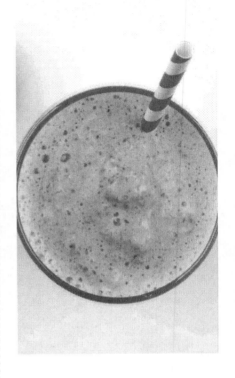

Caramel Coconut Cookie

1 scoop Chocolate IdealShake

1 c. unswt coconut milk

¾ c. low fat cottage cheese

¼ t. coconut extract

2 T. sugar free caramel syrup ice cream

1 T. sugar free chocolate syrup ice cream

2 T. oats

1 T. coconut oil, melted*

1 T. coconut flakes

Ice Cubes

Melt the coconut oil and then drizzle slowly into shake while blender is mixing to prevent clumping.

Berries n Cream

1 scoop Strawberry IdealShake

1 c. unswt almond milk

1 c. fat free plain greek yogurt

½ c. frozen raspberries

½ c. frozen strawberries

2 T. sugar free french vanilla creamer

1 T. fat free sugar free vanilla pudding mix

¼ c. oats

2 T. flax seeds

⅓ avocado

Ice Cubes

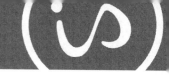

1 IdealBoost Stick Pack drink on the side with your snack!

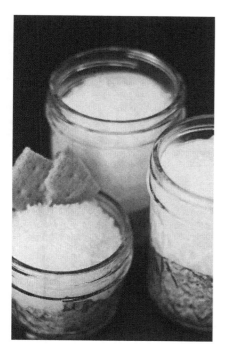

Coconut Cream Pie

1 container Coconut Chobani Greek yogurt

2 low fat graham cracker, crumbled

*Stir graham cracker crumbs into yogurt.

Easy Cheesecake

½ c. plain fat free Greek yogurt

½ c. low fat cottage cheese

2 T. sugar free cheesecake pudding powder

1 c. plain cheerios

*Sautee the cheerios on a pan over medium heat with spray butter and salt. Stir often. When they're lightly toasted cool in a bowl.

*Stir stevia and pudding powder into the Greek yogurt.

*Top the yogurt with the cheerios and enjoy!

Berries 'n' Cream

1 c. low fat cottage cheese

1 c. strawberries

Cinnamon and stevia, to taste

*Stir berries into cottage cheese and top with cinnamon and stevia

Fruit and Eggs

1 ½ c. grapes

2 hardboiled eggs

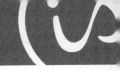

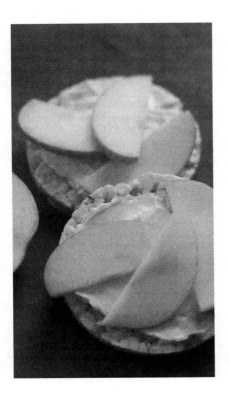

Apple Swiss Rice Cakes

2 wedges light *Laughing Cow* cheese

⅓ c. low fat cottage cheese

1 small granny smith apple, thinly sliced

2 lightly salted rice cakes

Spread the cheese over the rice cake and top with apple slices

Cheese and Crackers

1 serving whole wheat crackers

2 string cheese sticks

Turkey Sandwich

2 slices low carb 45 cal Sara Lee bread

4 oz turkey

½ T. light mayo

Lettuce, tomato, onion

Make a turkey sandwich and add lettuce tomato and onion

Fruit and Jerky

1 banana

2 oz beef jerky

Cheesy Rice Cake Snack

2 cheddar rice cakes

¾ c. low fat cottage cheese

Top the rice cake with cottage cheese

Cheesy Rice Cake Snack

2 cheddar rice cakes

¾ c. low fat cottage cheese

Top the rice cake with cottage cheese

Tuna "Sandwich"

3 oz tuna

1 hard boiled egg

½ T. light mayo

2 lightly salted rice cakes

Mix tuna and mayo and spread over the rice cake. Have egg on the side or mix into the tuna salad.

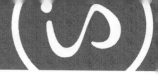

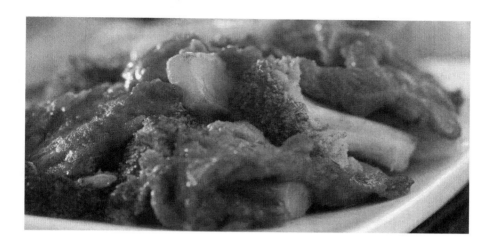

Beef and Broccoli Stir Fry

7 oz lean beef such as Top Sirloin, Flank or London Broil, sliced into thin slices

½ t. minced garlic

¼ t. ginger

½ T. light soy sauce

1 c. broccoli

½ T. coconut oil

2 T. water

6 T. beef broth

½ T. cornstarch

¼ c. bean sprouts, optional

2 T. peanuts, chopped

1 c. brown rice, cooked

1. Combine beef, garlic, ginger and soy sauce in a bowl and let stand.

2. Wash broccoli thoroughly and cut into florets.

3. Heat 1 t. oil in a nonstick skillet over high heat, add broccoli and stir fry for 2 minutes. Add water and stir until the water evaporates. Move broccoli to a separate bowl.

4. Heat remaining 2 t. oil, and add beef mixture. Stir fry for 3 minutes. Stir together broth and cornstarch, add to meat and stir fry until sauce is thickened, about 3 more minutes.

5. Add broccoli and bean sprouts, then cook, stirring, until heated through, about 2 more minutes.

6. Top with 2 T. chopped peanuts, spread over 1 c. brown rice and enjoy!

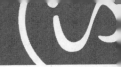

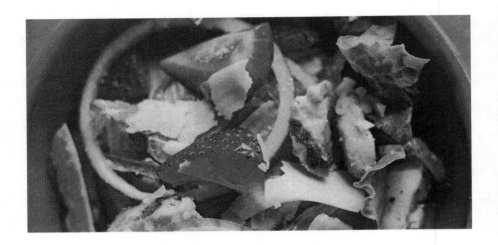

Maple Chicken Salad

Salad:

7 oz chicken, cooked and cut into strips

Romaine Lettuce

Red onion, thinly sliced

5 large strawberries

1 oz swiss cheese, shredded

2 slices turkey bacon, cooked and crumbled

1 c. quinoa, cooked

Dressing:

½ T. extra virgin olive oil

1 T. vinegar

½ T. light mayo

½ T. sugar free maple syrup

4 pecans, chopped, optional

Stevia to taste, if needed

1. *Combine dressing ingredients and allow to sit for 15-30 minutes in the fridge.*

2. *Meanwhile combine salad ingredients.*

3. *Toss salad in dressing and enjoy!*

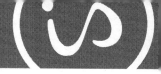

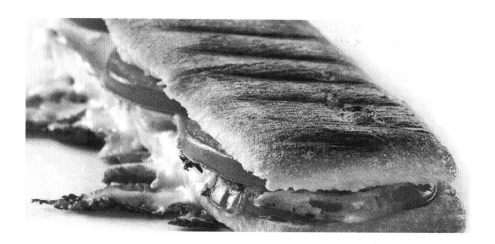

Balsamic Chicken Panini

8 oz chicken

½ c. Balsamic Vinegar

Whole bell pepper, thinly sliced

Sweet onion, thinly sliced

⅓ avocado, sliced

1 oz provolone cheese, sliced

1 Focaccia roll (approx 200 calories)

1. *Slice chicken breast in half so that it's cut thinly. Sautee in ¼ c. vinegar until cooked through.*

2. *Place chicken in a separate bowl. Sautee peppers and onion in ¼ c. vinegar until soft and cooked through.*

3. *Spray both sides of the sandwich thin with spray butter and assemble sandwich with chicken, veggies, avocado and cheese.*

4. *Grill the sandwich on an indoor grill (ie George Foreman) or on the stove in a pan over medium heat.*

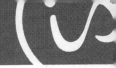

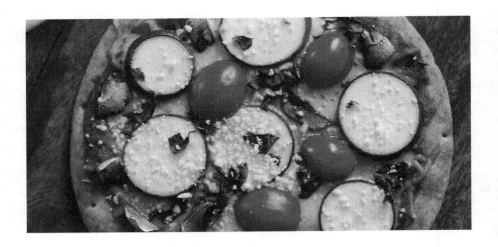

Low Carb Grilled Chicken Pizza

1 zucchini, thinly sliced

4 mushrooms, sliced

2 pitas or whole wheat tortillas
(approx 200 calories)

¼ c. tomato basil pizza sauce

3 oz low fat mozzarella cheese

4 cherry tomatoes

8 oz chicken, cooked and sliced

1 T. fresh basil, chopped

1. *Preheat ovent to 180 degrees.*

2. *Grill or roast zucchini and mushrooms until desired tenderness.* Transfer to a plate.*

3. *Place tortillas on a baking tray lined with foil. Spread sauce over tortillas and sprinkle with 3 oz of cheese. Top with grilled veggies, tomatoes*

and chicken. Top with remaining cheese.

4. *Bake for 12-15 minutes or until tortilla is crisp and cheese is melted. Sprinkle with basil and serve with a side salad.*

*To grill veggies preheat gas grill over medium heat. Spray the veggies with spray butter or cooking spray and lightly salt them. Cook over low-med heat for approx 5-8 minutes or until desired tenderness is reached. To roast veggies preheat oven to 400 degrees and bake on a baking sheet for approx 20-25 minute or until desired tenderness is reached. Then let oven cool before baking pizza.

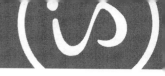

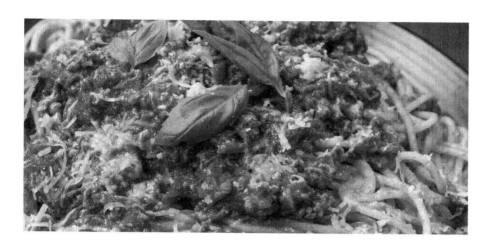

Creamy Bolognese over Spaghetti

¼ yellow onion, chopped

½ clove garlic

6 oz extra lean ground beef

½ c. premade spaghetti sauce

¼ can (14 oz) diced tomatoes, undrained

1 T. Light Italian Salad Dressing

1 T. fat free cream cheese

¼ t. dried basil

1 ½ oz whole wheat spaghetti noodles, dry

2 oz fresh Parmesan cheese

1. Sautee onions in a large skillet on medium heat until they begin to be translucent. Add meat and cook until cooked through, stirring frequently. Drain any excess grease from pan.

2. Meanwhile cook spaghetti noodles.

3. Stir in spaghetti sauce and tomatoes. Bring to a boil. Reduce heat to medium-low and simmer 15 minutes. Remove from heat and stir in cream cheese, seasonings and Italian salad dressing. Serve hot over cooked spaghetti squash noodles. Top with parmesan cheese.

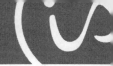

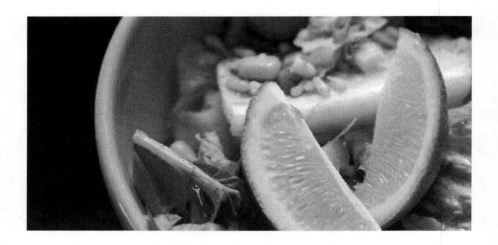

Garlic Lime Chicken Salad

3 T. low sodium soy sauce

1 T. lime juice

2 t. Worcestershire sauce

1 clove garlic

½ t. dry mustard

½ t. pepper

8 oz Chicken breast

1-2 cups romaine lettuce, chopped

Green onion, diced

¼ c. Corn

5 Cherry tomatoes, halved

¼ c. Peas

1 stick celery, diced

2 oz feta cheese

¾ c. brown rice

1. *Combine the first six ingredients for your sauce. Reserve 1 T. of the sauce for salad dressing.*

2. *Marinate chicken in the rest of the sauce for 15-30 minutes and grill.*

3. *Meanwhile assemble salad ingredients. Toss salad with rice, veggies, cheese and reserved sauce. Top with chicken.*

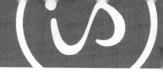

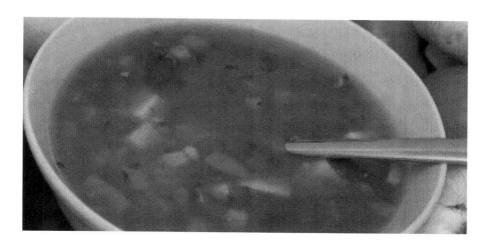

Vegetable, Beef and Barley Stew

7 oz extra lean ground beef

½ can (14.5 oz) stewed tomatoes, undrained, cut up

½ (14 oz) can beef broth

½ can (8 oz) no salt added tomato sauce

1 c. frozen mixed veggies

6 T. quick cooking barley

⅔ avocado, diced

1. *Brown ground beef and drain. In saucepan combine all ingredients and heat to boiling. Reduce heat to medium. Cover and cook 10-15 minutes, stirring occasionally until vegetables and barley are tender. Top with avocado.*

185

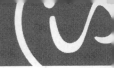

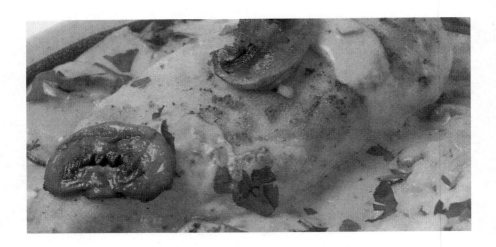

Creamy Crock Pot Chicken

7 oz Chicken breast

½ can cream of chicken soup

4 Sliced mushrooms

½ garlic cloves, pressed

¼ t. Worcestershire sauce

¼ t. lemon juice

1 slice turkey bacon, cooked and
crumbled

¼ t. vinegar

1 ½ oz cheddar cheese

1 c. white rice, prepared

1. Combine all ingredients except cheese, rice and chicken breast in a mixing bowl and mix well.

2. Put chicken into a crock pot. Cover with soup mixture.

3. Cook on low 4-6 hours or until cooked through.

4. While still hot top with shredded cheese and allow to melt. Serve with 1 c. white rice and steamed veggies.

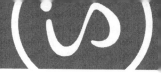

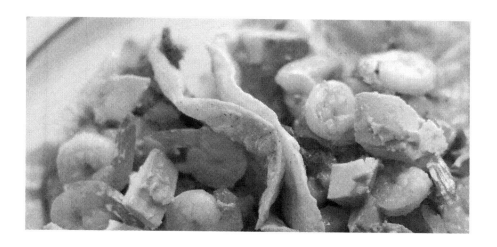

Honey Lime Shrimp Tacos

3 Corn Tortilla

8 oz Shrimp

½ Mango

1-2 cups chopped cabbage

Cilantro

Red Onion

2 t. Honey

1 lime

½ Avocado

1 t. coconut oil

1. *Warm your pan over medium heat and toast corn tortilla until it's slightly crispy.*

2. *Add 1 t. coconut oil to the pan and cook shrimp for 2-3 minutes.*

3. *Drizzle honey and squeeze the juice of half a lime onto the shrimp. Cook for another 3-4 minutes or until cooked through.*

4. *Meanwhile, dice mango and red onion and chop cilantro.*

5. *Assemble tacos drizzling the sauce over the shrimp. Top with cabbage, mango, onion and avocado.*

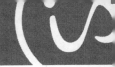

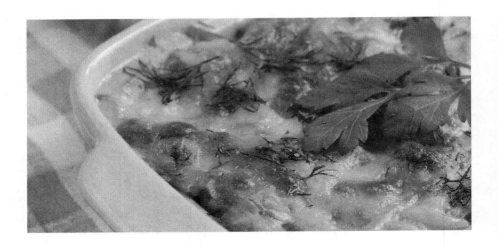

English Muffin Casserole

2 turkey sausage

2 whole wheat English muffins

1 oz low fat mozzarella cheese, shredded

1 oz low fat cheddar cheese, shredded

1 T. chopped onion

1 T. chopped bell pepper

2 eggs

¼ c. egg beaters

¼ c. milk

Salt and pepper to taste

1 slice turkey bacon

1. Cook sausage according to package directions. Cool slightly and cut into slices.

2. Cut English muffin into 1 inch cubes and put in greased single serving baking dish.

3. Layer with sausage, cheese, onion and bell pepper.

4. In a separate bowl combine eggs, milk, salt and pepper. Pour over the sausage and cheese mixture.

5. Top with crumbled bacon. Cover and refrigerate overnight.

6. Remove from the fridge 30 minutes prior to baking. Uncover and bake at 350 degrees for about 30 minutes or until a toothpick inserted in the center comes out clean. Let stand for 5 minutes before eating.

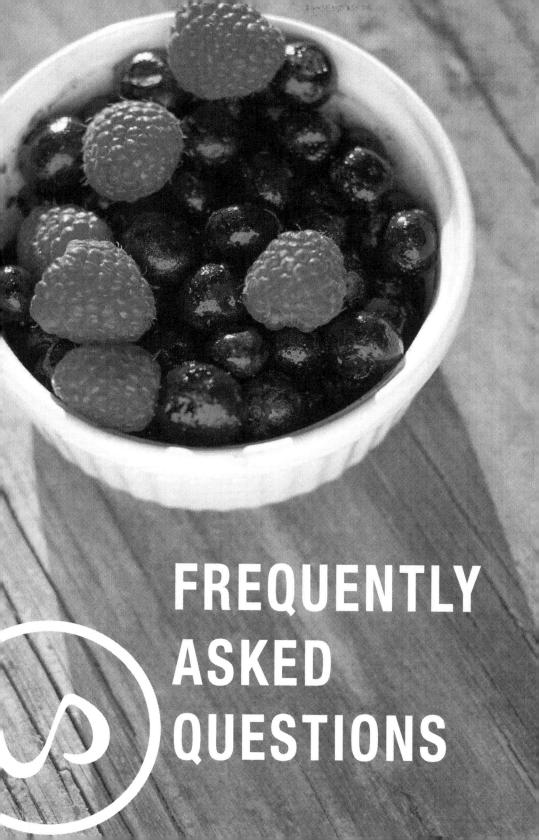

FREQUENTLY ASKED QUESTIONS

WHAT TO EXPECT

The key piece missing in every other weight loss meal plan is hunger control. And we'll say it again: if you can't control your hunger, you can't lose weight. By following the IdealPlan, you will be empowered to reduce calories, feel satisfied between meals, stay in control of your food choices, and ultimately change your appetite!

How Were the Calories, Portions and Foods on the IdealPlan Determined?

The meal plans are based on the average BMR (Basal Metabolic Rate) for each weight group. Your BMR is an estimate of how many calories you burn completely at rest (as in, laying in bed all day). Because we know you'll be active for at least some part of your day, you will be creating the calorie deficit necessary to lose weight. When you reach the point where you're ready to maintain your results, you can increase your calories above your BMR.

The foods we've chosen for your meals and snacks give you the ideal proportion of macronutrients (proteins, carbs and fats) to simultaneously fill you up and help your body shed fat and build lean muscle.

What Results Should You Expect?

Weight loss will vary from person to person, but a common, healthy and sustainable weight loss range is 1-2 pounds a week. Of course, the scale isn't the be-all-end-all for tracking progress. Weight can fluctuate from day to day for a variety of reasons, so in addition to tracking your weight, make sure to track your measurements and take progress pictures at each "Check-in" point. You can also choose a pair of tight jeans to try on every week. They won't be tight for long!

The 12-Week Timeline

Just like having a clear-cut plan helps you stay focused, so does setting a specific timeframe for your goals. We chose 12 weeks for the IdealPlan because it's long enough to kick-start your fat loss and see noticeable results, yet not so long that it feels like what you do today won't matter.

Once you finish your first 12-week round, you can set new goals in your IdealMind workbook and start again. You might even be ready to bump down to the next weight category!

Making This "Your" Plan

As you've probably guessed, every body is different! Furthermore, everyone has a different lifestyle and physical activity level. The "Check-in" points outlined below are great times to assess your results and adjust your meal plan as needed.

Phase 1 (Weeks 1-4)

Follow Phase 1 Accelerators at the end of Week 4, track your results in the IdealMind workbook and adjust your meal plan as needed using the guide below.

Phase 2 (Weeks 5-8)

Add Phase 2 Accelerators at the end of Week 8, track your results in the IdealMind workbook and adjust your meal plan as needed using the guide below. If you're following IdealBody, move on to Phase 2 of the workout program!

Phase 3 (Weeks 9-12)

Add Phase 3 Accelerators at the end of Week 12, track your results in the IdealMind workbook, adjust your meal plan as needed, and start the Plan again! If you're following IdealBody, move on to Phase 3 of the workout program!

How to Adjust Your Plan

Try any adjustment you make for 10 to 14 days. Because hormones change and weight can fluctuate for a variety of reasons, at least 10 days is needed to accurately assess whether a change is working for you.

If you're not seeing results...

The calories for each plan are approximate and there is a little wiggle room, because it depends on which foods you choose from the lists. So first, evaluate your food choices and choose the lower- calorie options from each list (e.g., switch cow's milk for almond milk, switch red meat for chicken, etc.). Try this for two weeks. If this doesn't work, then cut your dinner carb in half. Do this for two weeks and then reevaluate.

(Note: the "Women Under 140" meal plan doesn't have a dinner carb; however, this meal plan is approximately 1200 calories and we don't want you to cut your calories lower than this. It would be better to add two 20-minute cardio sessions to your week.)

If you've tried the above solutions and you're not seeing results, jump down to the next lower meal plan, try it for another two weeks and then reevaluate. If you still aren't seeing results, don't cut calories further; instead pay closer attention to things like BLTs ("bites, licks and tastes") and accurate food measurements to ensure that you're not having too much food without realizing it.

If you're still hungry...

When you begin a new diet not only do you have to learn and adjust to true hunger signals, your brain has to adjust to the amount of calories you are now consuming. Whenever I reduce my calories to reach a fitness goal, I usually have to battle hunger for about 7-10 days while my metabolism is adjusting, then that hunger goes away and I feel content and satisfied again.

If you find yourself battling hunger, try this: snack on fiber-rich "freebie" veggies listed in your meal plan, chew some gum, go outside and take a walk, or drink an IdealBoost to manage cravings/hunger. Also make sure you're drinking enough water. Sometimes when we think we're hungry we're actually dehydrated. Sip a big glass of water, wait 20 minutes and then decide how you feel.

If you still consistently feel hungry after 7-10 days and you're losing weight rapidly, you can add more healthy calories by jumping up to the next higher meal plan.

If you're too full...

If you feel too full to eat all of your meals as outlined in the plan, try sticking with it and eating all of the food for 7-10 days to see if it gets better. Often people have a slow metabolism when they first start a weight loss plan, but if you feed it enough it will actually speed up and that's a good thing! If after 7-10 days you're still overly full but you've lost a few pounds, stick with it and be thankful for the fullness because it means you aren't hungry. If you're still full and not losing any weight, then see suggestions above in the "I'm not seeing results" section.

F.A.Q.

Q **Can I Really Lose Weight By Eating Five Meals a Day?**

A The biggest barrier to fat loss is eating too much of the wrong foods. We know that controlling hunger and cravings is the hardest part of losing weight, so we've created a plan that helps you avoid "hunger triggers" by eating more often. On the IdealPlan, you'll have five small, healthy meals per day (and nothing in between) — not just any meals, but the specific hunger blocking foods we've outlined in the plan. By controlling cravings and avoiding the hunger danger zone with five daily means, you'll actually eat fewer calories overall!

Q **How Do You Know the IdealPlan Works?**

A We've drawn from scores of proven research from nutrition scientists and health behavior scholars to develop the principles and the right combination of hunger-blocking nutrients in this plan. Then we tested it for ourselves with men and women who had anywhere from 20 to more than 100 pounds to lose. It's effective because it curbs your hunger and creates a calorie deficit, while delivering the nourishment you need in a way that's sustainable and enjoyable, so you'll actually stick to it.

Q **Where Do I Get IdealBody and IdealMind?**

A The exercise program and goalsetting workbook should have come with your IdealPlan PDF, delivered via shopping cart download or sent to your email. If you didn't receive these e-books with your order, please contact customer service.

Q **Do I Need IdealShake, IdealBars and IdealBoost?**

A You can apply some of the principles we've shared with you and see some weight loss success. However, the IdealPlan is designed for maximum and lasting results, and IdealShake is an integral part of the program. IdealBars and IdealBoost are optional, but they will enhance your results. Our products contain a powerful hunger-blocking formula, are low-calorie, and give people the convenience and simplicity to choose healthy every day.

Q **How Many Shakes and Bars Can I Have Each Day?**

A Replace up to 2 of your 5 meals with an IdealShake and 1 snack with IdealBar each day, as outlined in the IdealPlan. Your other meals are outlined for you in the meal plan.

Q **What If I Want to Have a Shake or Bar for Dessert in the Evening?**

A Lots of people like to have an IdealShake or IdealBar for dessert. To stick to your calorie goal, you can rearrange your meals in this order: shake, snack, snack, dinner, shake. You can also space your meals a little farther apart.

Q **What are the Shake Instructions?**

A You'll add one scoop of IdealShake to 8oz of a liquid of your choice (water or one of the options in the milk list). Shake the mixture in the IdealShape shaker bottle that is included, or use your electric blender, and enjoy! Follow your shake with an additional 8oz of water to activate the shake's full hunger blocking potential.

Q **Does IdealShake Contain Caffeine or Other Stimulants?**

A The Chocolate and Mocha IdealShake flavors contain a very small amount of caffeine from cocoa beans. Chocolate IdealShake contains 4g of cocoa, or roughly 0.4 mg caffeine per serving. Mocha IdealShake contains 2g of cocoa, or roughly 0.2 mg caffeine per serving. (As a reference point, a cup of coffee contains roughly 100mg of caffeine.) Vanilla and Strawberry IdealShake flavors contain no caffeine.

195

Q Is the IdealPlan Safe to Follow While Pregnant or Nursing?

A Aside from a very minimal amount of caffeine in the Chocolate and Mocha shake flavors, the IdealShake contains no caffeine or stimulants. The rest of the meals and snacks on the plan are stimulant free, with the exception of the optional IdealBoost drink. Using a meal replacement shake while pregnant or nursing may require including additional nutrients; the IdealPlan includes guidelines for adding healthy sources of each macronutrient to your shake. You may wish to include additional nutrients or increase your calorie goals. We always advise our customers who are pregnant or nursing to consult with their physician before using our products.

Q What If It Doesn't Work for Me?

A We offer a 100% risk free money- back guarantee for 30 days if for any reason you're not satisfied. That's because we're confident that the IdealPlan program and IdealShape products are the most powerful way to shed fat!

Still Have a Question?

Do you have another question about our products or your experience using the IdealPlan? Contact our customer service team and we'll be glad to help!

(800) 515-0896
customerservice@idealshape.com

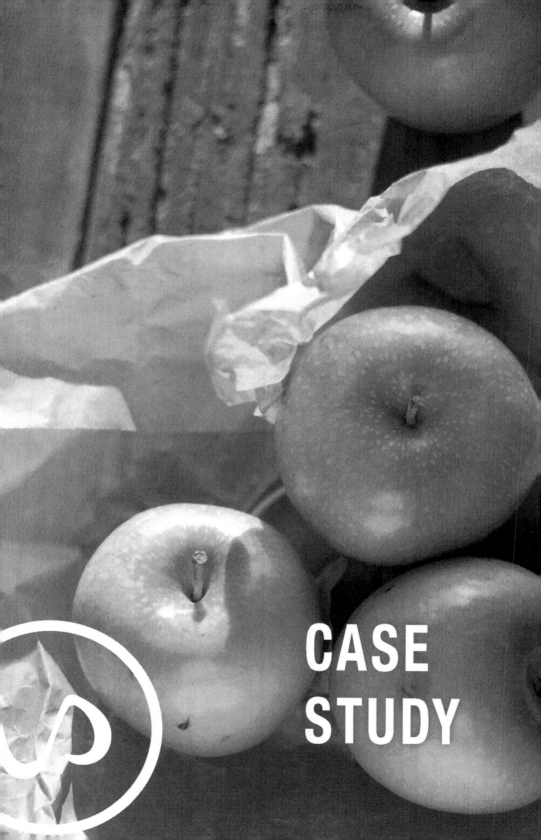

CASE
STUDY

IDEALPLAN CASE STUDY

USE OF MEAL REPLACEMENT SHAKES AND EATING FIVE MEALS A DAY IN APPETITE CONTROL AND WEIGHT LOSS

Conducted by Lindsey Mathews, IdealShape Nutritionist, and Whitney Meine, IdealShape Product Manager

ISSUE

Appetite control is one of the biggest problems when it comes to weight loss. When a person is trying to change eating habits, reduce calorie intake, and start making smart food choices they have a lot to adapt to. They are used to taking in an uncontrolled amount of calories. The human body becomes persistent at keeping the bad habits formed from eating at random times, and in most cases people think they are hungry even when they are not. Adding a type of appetite control or hunger blocker through a meal replacement shake to a diet could keep people from overeating throughout the day. Also, eating five smaller meals throughout the day may help

control cravings and curb appetite allowing for greater weight loss. The number one meal that has been shown to help control appetite is breakfast. Having no breakfast meal at all has been known to increase overeating, gaining weight and obesity (Leidy & Racki, 2010).

OVERVIEW

The importance of satiety is common in a lot of studies (Veldhorst & Hochstenbach-Waelen, 2009; Rothacker & Watemberg, 2004; Leidy & Racki, 2010; Weigle et al., 2005). Studies have shown that appetite control can lead to prevention of obesity and aid in weight loss (Leidy et al., 2010). Satiety is critical to the success with any weight loss plan or diet (Rothacker et al., 2004). Satiety affects not only just the period of time between meals before feeling hunger, but also the amount of food that is consumed in the next meal (Benelam, 2009). The best meal to support appetite control is breakfast. Studies done on breakfast meals affect the appetite by lowering appetite levels and decreasing the need for calorie rich foods throughout the day (Leidy et al., 2010). Increased eating frequency has also been shown to improve appetite control and subsequent fat loss (Munsters & Saris, 2012).

CONSIDERATIONS

Although appetite control aids in weight loss and prevention of obesity, studies have yet to find one specific food that works best. Meal replacement shakes with or without an added hunger blocker may not work for everyone and not a lot of studies have been done with meal replacement shakes specifically. Appetite control is also dependent on individual characteristics, including unhealthy eating habits they may have integrated into their lives over time. For example, individuals may eat even if they don't have the feeling of hunger.

PURPOSE

The purpose of this study is to find out whether eating five meals a day and using meal replacements with hunger control (specifically, replacing two of the five meals with a hunger-blocking meal replacement shake and one of the five meals with a hunger-blocking snack bar) will help individuals control appetite and lose weight more effectively compared with their prior dieting experiences.

HYPOTHESIS

It is hypothesized that those who have meal replacement shakes/bars with an added hunger blocker and eat five small meals a day will have a more controlled appetite and will lose more weight than those who do not use these products or follow a meal plan with five meals a day.

SIGNIFICANCE

Although having a meal replacement shake with a hunger blocker first thing in the morning could increase appetite control, not a lot of studies have specifically studied the relationship of meal replacement shakes with a hunger blocker and the effects on appetite control. This study will help show if meal replacement shakes are sufficient for appetite control along with the habit of eating five small meals a day thereby controlling hunger leading to weight reduction.

METHODS

A sample of 21 individuals (18 women and 3 men) ages 25-60, with 20 or more pounds to lose, participated in this 12-week study. Prior to beginning the program, participants provided their starting weight and measurements (chest, waist, glutes, right thigh, right calf, right arm).

During the program, participants completed weekly check-in's reporting their weight and measurements, and whether they complied with the plan for that week. They also reported their hunger, energy, and sleep levels. They also participated in a forum-style Facebook group where they could ask questions and post their progress.

Participants were given IdealShake hunger-blocking meal replacement shake mix and IdealBar hunger-blocking snack bars. They were instructed to follow a meal plan provided, which outlined five small daily meals/snacks.

The plan included two meal replacement shakes (one for breakfast and one for lunch) and one IdealBar as a snack. For the other two meals, participants had a whole food snack and a whole food dinner from the food lists and recipes in the meal plan.

Participants were instructed to follow a meal plan for their specific weight range. Meal plans were divided into the following five weight categories, designed to create a calorie deficit conducive to effective, healthy weight loss:

Women under 140 pounds: 1,200 calories

Women 140-190 pounds: 1,500 calories

Women 190 pounds and above: 1,800 calories

Men under 250 pounds: 2,000 calories

Men over 250 pounds: 2,200 calories

Participants were instructed to add ingredients to the shakes from the food lists (or comparable foods) in order to achieve roughly the target calorie amount and an optimum balance of macronutrients (roughly 40/30/30 carbs, fats and proteins).

The plan included one "cheat meal" per week, for which participants could eat anything they wanted. This was done to allow participants to occasionally enjoy their favorite foods and not feel restricted on the diet.

Participants were instructed to time their five daily meals roughly three hours apart.

RESULTS

All program participants (21) completed the study and lost weight. In 12 weeks, each participant lost between 9-40 pounds, with an average of 17 pounds per person. Each participant lost between 6-36 inches, with an average of 15 inches per person.

Although exercise was not part of the program, 15 participants performed some level of physical activity during the 12-week period, while 6 people did not.

More than three-fourths (78%) of participants followed at least 7 of the Accelerators outlined in the book for the duration of the program.

PARTICIPANT FEEDBACK

Participants were invited to complete an online survey after the study concluded. When asked what they felt helped them most to comply with the program, 94% of participants said it was because "the plan was complete and 'done for you' so I didn't have to think about what and when to eat." Additionally, 61% said "the plan helped me to manage hunger and cravings."

Following along with other participants on social media was moderately important, and how well the plan fit with their daily lifestyle and food preferences was ranked low in importance.

REFERENCES

Benelam B. (2009) Satiation, satiety and their effects on eating behavior. *Nutrition bulletin,* 34(2), 126-173

HJ Leidy, EM Racki. (2010). The addition of a protein-rich breakfast and its effects on acute appetite control and food intake in 'breakfast-skipping' adolescents.

Arazi, H., Benar, N., Esfanjani, R.M., & Yeganegi, S. (2012). The effect of an aerobic training on perceived stress. *International journal of Obesity.* 34 11251133

Munsters MJ, Saris WH. (2012) Effects of meal frequency on metabolic profiles and substrate partitioning in lean healthy males. *PLoS One,* 7(6)

Rothacker Dana Q,,Watemberg Salo. (2004) Short-Term

Hunger Intensity Changes Following Ingestion of A Meal Replacement Bar for Weight Control. *International Journal of Food Properties. 7, 553-559*

Veldhorst V.,Nieuwenhuizen A., Hochstenbach-Waelen A. (2009) Effects of complete whey-Protein Areak- fasts versus whey without GMP-breakfasts on energy intake and satiety. *Appetite,* 52(3), 388-395

Weigle D.S, Breen P.A, Matthys C.C., Callahan H.S.,

Meeuws K.E., Burden V.R, & Purnell, J.Q. (2005)

A high-protein diet induces sustained reductions in appetite, and libitum caloric intake, and body weight despite compensatory changes in diurnal plasma leptin and ghrelin concentrations. *American Journal of Clinical Nutrition,* 82, 41-48

TESTIMONIALS

"Great program and very helpful. The plan was laid out like you were talking to us one to one."

"At first I felt overwhelmed because there was so much info but after a week it was one of easiest diets that I have ever been on!"

"It helped me learn my body's hunger signals, and taught me to use that as a guide. I liked eating three hours apart because I was hungry for each meal, but not starving."

"It was hard to wrap my mind around the concept of eating more to lose weight...but it's true!"

"I didn't eat that much before, but I was surprised at how little I really needed. Eating the right food at 3-hour intervals and drinking water made such a difference."

"Watching calories made me realize how much sugar and fat really are in the foods I had been eating."

"I learned a lot about macronutrients that I didn't know much about before. It gave me a foundation for doing further research online to understand even more."

"Just eating more often helped. I used to not eat all day thinking I would lose weight but never did."

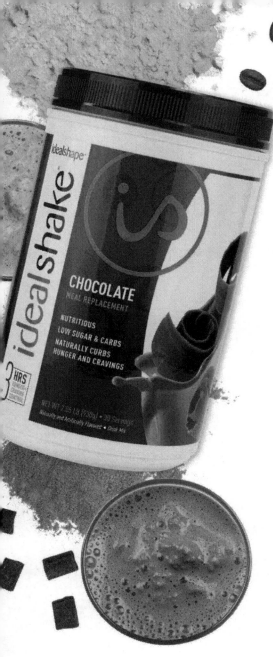

IdealShake®

Available in Chocolate, Vanilla, Strawberry, and Mocha High Quality Protein Blend

High Quality Protein Blend

A protein-rich diet is essential to fat loss, but it's hard to get enough of it without adding excess calories, sugars and fats. A quality protein supplement is an excellent aid in maintaining lean, healthy muscle and burning calories more efficiently.

Balanced Nutrition

IdealShake has 11 grams of protein per serving and over 40% of your recommended daily intake (RDI) of 22 vitamins and minerals.

Hunger Blocker

If you can't control your hunger, you can't lose weight. Our shake puts you in control with the all-natural hunger blocker Slendesta. Slendesta is proven to help you feel full for up to 3 hours by triggering the release of CCK, a hormone that tells your brain when you're full.

Low Calories

Each shake contains only 100 calories per serving. It's filling and delicious by itself, yet low-calorie enough to make a perfect base for smoothies

Low Sugar

Refined sugar is a major contributing factor to diabetes, obesity and numerous chronic diseases. IdealShake is sweetened with sucralose, so it satisfies your sweet tooth with only 1 gram of sugar per serving.

High Fiber

With 5 grams of fiber per serving, IdealShake will help you get the fiber you need in your diet to improve digestion and weight loss by moving calories throughout your body without being absorbed.

Buy now at *www.idealshape.com*

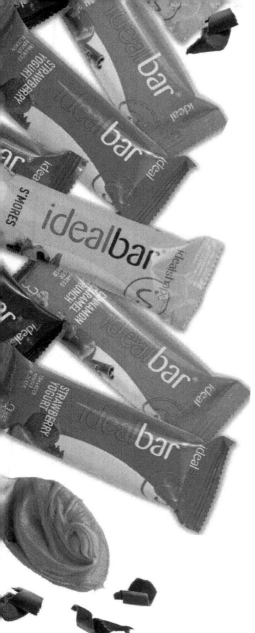

IdealBar® Snack Bar

Available in Chocolate Peanut Butter, Cinnamon Caramel Crunch, Double Chocolate, Strawberry Yogurt and S'mores

High Quality Protein Blend

A quality protein bar makes the perfect midday snack. IdealBar delivers 10 grams of protein, helping you get more protein in your diet while keeping you feeling full longer.

Balanced Nutrition

IdealBar has 10 grams of protein per bar and 20% of your recommended daily intake (RDI) of 24 vitamins and minerals. All in a low-fat, 140-calorie snack that's convenient for on the go!

Hunger Blocker

Unlike snacks that whet your appetite for more sugar or salt, IdealBars contain the power of the all-natural hunger blocker Slendesta® to help you feel satisfied for up to 3 hours.

Low Sugar

Each flavor of IdealBar contains only 6-8 grams of sugar, delighting your sweet tooth while keeping sugar content much lower than other commercial snacks.

High Fiber

With 5 grams of fiber per serving, IdealBar will keep you feeling full, while helping to improve digestion and weight loss.

Buy now at *www.idealshape.com*

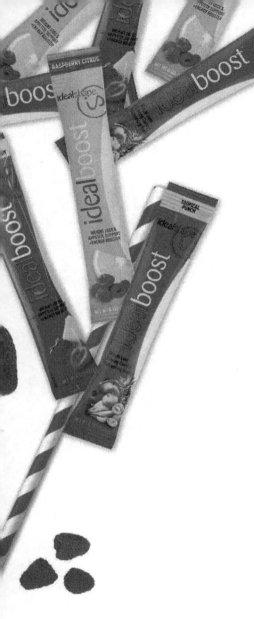

IdealBoost® Drink Mix

Available in Raspberry Citrus, Pineapple Strawberry, and Tropical Punch

Energy Boost

With a combination of green tea, green coffee bean and caffeine anhydrous, IdealBoost contains 80mg of caffeine, about the same amount of caffeine as a cup of coffee for an anytime pick-me-up.

Fat-Blasting Benefits

The real benefit of IdealBoost is in the power combo of green tea and caffeine. Both are proven aids in boosting metabolism and helping the body convert fat into energy. Research has found that green tea-caffeine consumption can help people achieve reduced body weight, waist size and body fat.

Immunity Boost

IdealBoost contains vitamins B3, B6 and B12, which contribute to healthy cell function, improving everything from skin to metabolism to mood. Green tea provides extra support with antioxidant and anti-inflammatory properties to help the body fight disease.

Hunger Blocker

Slendesta® is an all-natural hunger blocker that helps you feel full for up to 3 hours, so you stay in control of your cravings between meals. And for an extra boost, IdealBoost contains Fibersol, a soluble dietary fiber, to decrease hunger and aid in healthy digestion and regularity.

Low Calories & Sugar

Each stick pack contains only 5 calories and 0 grams of sugar, making it a delicious yet totally guilt-free drink!

Buy now at *www.idealshape.com*

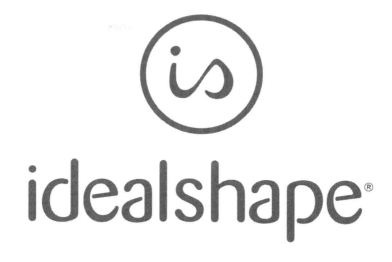

idealshape®

#CHANGE*YOUR*APPETITE

ALL RIGHTS RESERVED © IDEALSHAPE, LLC
2015 American Fork, UT 84003

800-515-0896

24871498R00121

Made in the USA
San Bernardino, CA
10 October 2015